Bodybuilding at Home

Building a Complete Home Gym

A Step By Step Guide

Craig Cecil

Bodybuilding at Home
Building a Complete Home Gym,
A Step By Step Guide

ISBN: 978-0-9847414-6-5

ISBN: 978-0-9847414-7-2 (ebook)

First edition: October 2015

Manufactured in the United States of America

Trademarked names may appear in this book. Rather than use a trademark symbol with every occurrence of a trademarked name, we use the names only in an editorial fashion and to the benefit of the trademark owner, with no intention of infringement of the trademark.

Warning: This book stresses the importance of proper technique and safety when using bodybuilding and strength training programs. Regardless of your age, before beginning any exercise program consult with your physician to ensure that you are in proper health and that it is appropriate for you to follow such programs. Proceed with caution and at your own risk. This book does not provide medical or therapeutic advice; you should obtain medical advice from your healthcare practitioner. Before starting any new exercise program, check with your doctor, especially if you have a specific physical problem or are taking any medication. The author, publisher or distributors of this book cannot be responsible for any injury, loss or damage caused, or allegedly caused, directly or indirectly, from following the instruction given in this book.

Cover design by Jaclyn Urlahs.
Cover photo by Nikolay Suslov (NiDerLander).

This book is for all the guys who pushed, pulled, strained and bared their souls with me over the past quarter century. And most importantly, for just showing up—week after week, year after year. I've tried to immortalize as many of you as possible within these pages.

Thank you to Eric Uhland of InstaSigns (www.instasigns.net) for the great photography in this book.

A special thanks to the following training partners and friends who graciously offered to pose for some of the pictures: Andrew "Arms Like Jesus", Jake "The Original Chin Strap", Tyler, Jay "The Prototype", John "Mad Dog" Bosley, "Crazy" Matt, and Katherine ('Kit').

This book is also for Leslie, who now has the finest gym just beyond the laundry room door, and for Kayleigh, Alexa, and Julia, who watched their dad transform half of their garage into this strange place with mirrors, weird apparatus and cast iron. Girls, the possibilities are endless...and the transformation is beyond the physical.

Contents

Home is where the heart is.

— Gaius Plinius Secundas

Once a man has made a commitment to a way of life, he puts the greatest strength in the world behind him. It's something we call heart power. Once a man has made this commitment, nothing will stop him short of success.

— Vince Lombardi

❶

Freedom & Purpose

My uncle Ray was a rugged outdoorsman, raised in the Appalachian mountains of western Maryland. I remember visiting him when I was a boy, wandering around his remote home and staring at the mounts of past adventures and the reflections of his craft. Deer, elk, and other conquests adorned the walls of his house and the high rafters of his spacious garage. A trained taxidermist and humble realist, Ray made use of every resource, including that garage. Part workshop, part smokehouse and a part I didn't yet understand. I remember staring at two things in particular that day—all the cast iron weights and my uncle's arms. Standing five foot seven and weighing almost two hundred pounds, dressed in cowboy boots, jeans that hugged the legs and a short-sleeved t-shirt tucked neatly at the waist—a shirt that barely contained those enormous arms. Arms immortalized in my memory. What I didn't realize until years later, is that he forged that forty three year old body—a body that won the Maryland State Bodybuilding Championship—right there in his garage gym.

A decade later, spurred on largely by that memorable day and those memorable arms, I started down a similar path. Initially, like most young men, I started lifting weights at home, eventually migrating to a commercial gym when I outgrew and out-lifted my meager equipment. However, I gained my first twenty pounds of muscle in that makeshift home gym, in a back room behind my parent's garage. I was hardly alone in this type of endeavor.

In the southeastern Alaska island city of Ketchikan, only accessible by boat or plane, another man made the daily, ritualized trek to his unheated backyard shed. After chipping away the ice that had accumulated on the bar in that unforgiving winter environment and loading on some cast iron plates, Dennis Weis began yet another grueling workout—one in a long

30-year tenure that would mold the Yukon Hercules into one of the legendary bodybuilders and powerlifters of the west coast. Necessity sometimes drives a man.

At eighty years old, five-time Mr. Universe Bill Pearl still rises at 2:30am each morning in Talent, Oregon, grabbing a hot cup of coffee and quick breakfast before walking briskly from the house to his converted barn to engage in another test against the weights—a test and testament that's been ongoing for over half a century. Pearl quickly asserts that he did most of his fundamental training and built the bulk of his award-winning physique in the nine years he spent in the basement gym at his parent's house.

At the turn of the century, while circus strongmen entertained with feats of strength and the era of physical culture was birthing, youth across America were getting stronger, leaner and more muscular in our original gym—the farm.

Today, much of the world lies to you.

You don't need state-of-the-art, modern equipment and machines to build muscle and transform yourself. You don't need a membership at a commercial gym. Let's take a look at this.

The number of health clubs in the U.S. has increased by more than 200% over the past 25 years, fueled by the growth of big-box facilities such as Planet Fitness, Golds Gym and L.A. Fitness, in addition to independent franchises such as Curves and CrossFit gyms. However, over the same period the increase in the number of overweight, obese, diabetic, and unhealthy individuals has grown significantly as well. If supply exists to accommodate demand, does that sound right? And what does that tell you about results?

While initially shiny and tempting, after succumbing to the New Year's siren song of change and opportunity, problems with commercial gyms become evident. These issues are legion and growing.

Foremost, commercial gyms sap your time. Time spent driving there, changing clothes, waiting on equipment. You already spend a large portion of your life just waiting. Waiting in traffic, in lines at the bank, grocery store, movie theater, etc. When you just calculate your travel time to and from the gym for a year, it's often eye-opening. With a home gym, that opportunity cost immediately goes to zero and you reclaim all that lost time into your life.

Second, commercial gyms try to fit you into their schema—their hours, their equipment, their rules—regardless of your schedule and your individual goals. In essence, you are effectively leasing their space and equipment within a cauldron of rules and people you may or may not like, in an attempt to improve in an environment not necessarily conducive to progress. A home gym flips this on its head, because your goals, your schedule, your resources and your wallet drive the whole operation. Your gym meets your specific goals. Commercial gyms offer shaky promises and hope. Home gyms demand it.

Third, and perhaps most insidious is what's actually happening in these gyms today. Steven Covey, among others, tells us in *The 7 Habits of Highly Effective People* that successful people study, emulate and extend what other successful people are doing. Success breeds success. Results breed results. Aspirations foster inspirations. Noted strength coach Pavel Tsatsouline (*Easy Strength*) tells us what he encountered:

"A few months ago, I trained at a gym once known for strength. Not anymore. The biggest "feat" I saw there was a 315 squat—by a guy who weighed about that much. It was a nose-bleed high squat, too...a dude was faking lunges...Horrified, I went to the corner and started deadlifting."

Sure, you can work out in similar environs, but chances are, especially if you are in the novice or intermediate stages of progress, your results may be restricted by emulating or being affected by the flagrant ignorance of the masses.

Furthering these illusions and restrictions, commercial gyms offer a landscape ripe for working out, and not for training. There is a big difference. Training, especially intermediate and advanced training requires a specific, planned execution of exercises, weight increments and rep schemes—programming—conducted over some predetermined period to affect the desired adaptation. It also requires concentration. That's something that commercial gyms, with their unpredictable influx of patrons cannot guarantee. They can, however, almost guarantee programmed failure. One day, the squat rack or all the benches might be occupied. Those dumbbells you were going to use for a back-off set are there—one of them. You've seen this. Home gyms guarantee a training environment. Just this difference, between working out and training, over an extended period, can have a dramatic effect on your physique.

The final damnation is the most obvious. Big-box gyms are built for the masses and mediocrity, tilting toward cardiovascular fitness, with standard floor configurations dominated with treadmills, bikes, rowers, steppers and any other cardio de jour equipment they may be offering. Beyond the cardio, low-load isolation machines line the floor. The free weights are relegated to the back, not unlike some lunch counter patrons in the deep south of 1960s America. Deadlifts and chalk are either discouraged or prohibited. Sweating is obscene and noise, such as grunting during heavy exertions, is offensive.

Almost a century ago, Ayn Rand wrote about a future where we have become the same—stripped of our individuality, thought, dreams and desire. A future hindering progress at every step. Today we call that Planet Fitness. As our society becomes increasingly restrictive, commercial gyms have mirrored this descent. Powerlifters have faced this stark reality for decades now. It's here that home gyms offer the libertarian solution—the le' resistance—to the marching boots of conformity and the assembly line of mediocrity. Resist the urge, free yourself and ascend to the true limitations of the physique that God gave you.

This is the clarion call. I hope you answer it.

• • • •

So, based on all you've read so far, we finally ask the most important question—what do the majority of people want to accomplish by "working out"?

I know the answer because I've witnessed it a thousand-fold over a quarter century.

You want to build some muscle, lose some fat, and in general, look a helluva lot better than you do right now. Well, ladies and gentlemen— that's called bodybuilding. We're not talking about the drug-addled physiques bulging from the bodybuilding magazines at the supermarket check-out line. Those are the outliers, the freaks and the cheats. No, what we are defining is the essence of the word itself—*bodybuilding*. To build the body into something greater. Often, that requires a concerted combination of fat loss and muscle building (hypertrophy), something that most find appealing and that represents the true fountain of youth.

So, where does the answer lie?

For many, it's right at home.

Now is the time to take a stand and make some decisions for yourself, instead of allowing others to dictate the arc and destination of your progress. As former judge Thomas Penfield Jackson noted, "When you discover you are riding a dead horse, the best strategy is to dismount." Let us venture back into our homes, garages or basements, not as hermits, but as part of a holistic approach to an intelligent, determined, and defined training regimen. Free yourself from commercial constraint and allow your physique to develop into the image you aspire to.

I've trained in commercial gyms for more than 25 years, as many of you have, so it may appear contradictory for someone like me to recommend the move to a home gym as a desirable alternative. However, if you take a moment to really look around, to remember how it used to be, you'll realize that the true gyms, the places you could always count on to transform yourself, these places are quickly disappearing. The era of the cast iron in the big-box, commercial gym is passing.

A home gym is freedom. The freedom to work out your way (think deadlifts), freedom to work out when you want and the freedom to help your kids work out, regardless of their age (the minimum age for membership in most commercials gyms is 13, due to perceived liability issues). Here, everyone in the family can become physically fit—no one is prohibited, regardless of age, time of day, geographic location or even income. Especially for kids, home gyms can really pick up where our government schools have failed us over the past decades in general physical preparedness (and the benefits can far surpass the physical). For others, like our Yukon Hercules, living in remote or less populated areas, a home gym may be the only alternative. Home gyms really are the worldwide workout—the great equalizer in the fitness equation. This combination of freedom and convenience can be a powerful motivator.

My home gym has allowed me, my wife and kids, and even occasional visiting relatives and friends to get productive, intense workouts at all hours of the day and night, on weekends and holidays, even during snowstorms. Throughout this book, I'll show and describe to you how I built, organized and extended mine over time.

At this point, you might be thinking, "I don't have the money, space or time to create my own gym." Wrong. As I'll explain, you can start with as little as $50—that's one or two month's membership dues at most gyms—and be ready to go in a day or two. From there, you'll see how to expand on that intelligently and systematically to provide more options and results.

Goals for this book

You can find lots of information in various books and magazines and on the Internet about setting up your own home gym. However, they tend to focus on outfitting a home gym for general fitness goals, powerlifting or CrossFit-type training, and lack substantive depth to the information. This book focuses on building a home gym for bodybuilding purposes and then showing you how to use it to maximum effect. To that end, it's hypertrophy and fat-burning focused and a mile deep in details.

This book also has some additional goals.

- To guide you through the process of assembling a home gym with the minimum amount of equipment that produces maximum results for bodybuilding purposes. We want the training trifecta here—combining safety, effectiveness and efficiency while minimizing space and cost. We're talking less equipment, more focus, and more efficient training. Here, less truly is more. For many, building an excellent training facility in a garage, basement or spare room is daunting. Strategic planning is the key here and this book will guide you through this process. Be smart about the location, layout, equipment and price. Combine all these aspects and you'll have friends asking when they can join "your gym".

- To make the workout safe and simple to do alone, regardless of the exercise or the amount of weight used. We want to avoid being pinned under bars and dropping barbells on your head. When obtaining equipment for the home gym, always err on the side of safety.

- To maximize the number and variety of bodybuilding exercises you can perform, given the constraints of location, space, and budget, while providing a stepwise approach that enables a systematic extension of what you have.

- To save you thousands of dollars by avoiding bad or sub-optimal purchases. The Chinese have a proverb for this—"One step in the wrong direction will cause you a thousand years of regret." Well, it might not be that bad, but you don't want to keep correcting for missteps. The equipment recommended in this book represents high quality, safe, and effective instruments of adaptation that will last a lifetime and won't lead you astray. Some of the equipment you should buy (new or used) and others you can make, if desired. If that sounds like you, I'll show you how. What is the payback period? Often, it's a moving target as your equipment costs climb. However, as I've mentioned the payback is immediate in time savings.

- To save you time. We've touched on family and relationships, so time is a precious commodity, often undervalued when you're young.

- To provide you with some solid bodybuilding workouts and training plans, regardless of your experience and adaptation level, that you can use immediately in your home gym *as you accumulate the equipment*. These workouts and training plans can take you from absolute beginner all the way to the competitive stage. One of my foremost goals for this book was not to leave you hanging, especially if you don't know how to train yourself. I don't want to just show you how to put this gym together and then say "you did it, now good luck". I want to provide you with the info to use it effectively. I'll try to light the fire—it's up to you to keep it burning.

- A final goal—and if you've read any of my other books, you know this—is to provide you with some history, because, well it's important, it helps put people, places and things in context and learning can be fun and it lets you show off to your friends.

I have a quarter century of experience with gyms, gym equipment, and bodybuilding training that I think will be instrumental in providing you with insight, monetary savings, and paving the road to success in home-based bodybuilding. With the systematic process in this book, you can build an excellent strength and conditioning facility in your home or on your property—one designed to get you stronger, build bigger muscles and a leaner body—transforming yourself in the process.

Let's get started.

❷

A Bodybuilder's Gym

Unlike the commercial, big-box gyms, a home gym distills the essence of physical transformation without drowning the truth in a sea of irrelevance. We need to strip away our infinite appetite for distractions—most of the machines and unnecessary apparatus—and get to the things that produce the most adaptation. Lucky for us, that saves a lot of money and space.

Someone once said that bodybuilders are just frustrated powerlifters—maybe so. However, all good bodybuilders, people who really know how to physically transform their appearance, start with a solid base in fundamental powerlifting movements. That means squats, deadlifts, rows and presses. Pushing, pulling, squatting and hinging. Training those basic human movements in a progressively overloaded environment requires a bare minimum of equipment and space—a barbell, some plates, a bench and a rack.

A powerlifter's gym is the essence of progress, following Pareto's Law where 80% of the results come from just 20% of the efforts (squats, deadlifts and presses using the rack, bench, bar and plates).

A *successful* bodybuilder's gym is a natural extension of a powerlifting gym, allowing the bodybuilder to start with Pareto and eventually progress to a 50/50 ratio of basic/accessory movements (but never abandoning the powerlifting core). While powerlifting focuses on a limited set of exercises, often with little to no direct cardio work, bodybuilding extends this baseline through derivatives of these core lifts, thus extending the equipment requirements as well. The training also differs.

A powerlifter is concerned with moving the most weight possible, hence the body operates as a unit. The bodybuilder, in contrast, has the additional concerns of maximizing muscular tissue size, ensuring muscular symmetry and reducing body fat. These added concerns require a complete overload and exhaustion of every muscle fiber type—attempting to coax, conjure, and shove the adaptive hypertrophic process. This requires time under tension, muscle isolation and apportioning of the body in order to maximize development of every facet. Over time, the seasoned bodybuilder, like any successful athlete, understands the importance of accumulation of movements, intensity, and allowing those things to transform their physique, all within a limited adaptive capacity. Eventually, every successful bodybuilder becomes concerned with not only strength, but toward the qualities of hypertrophy (size), shape, symmetry, muscular endurance and lean body mass.

These extended concerns—this accumulation of movements—lead to the need for some additional equipment.

Of course, we need the barbell and the plates. But the dumbbell rises in this pantheon of hypertrophy to new heights, and the importance of cables and their duality of constant tension and freedom of movement emerges as a major participant. The standard flat bench requires an inclined brother. Finally, we must concern ourselves with some type of cardio machine that we can perform indoors throughout all seasons and weather concerns, as necessary.

Therefore, to sum up, bodybuilders need a barbell, plates, dumbbells, an adjustable bench, a rack, some type of cable/pulley system and a piece of cardio equipment. We've just distilled 90% of the equipment in any commercial gym down to about six things. These six things will allow you to perform every essential (and even non-essential!) compound and isolation exercise devised in the bodybuilding universe. These tools will make the greatest impact. Everything else is just icing on the cake.

This final setup, occupying not much more space than the Spartan powerlifter's bench and rack, creates a maximum transformation chamber, optimized for compound, multi-joint movements affecting entire muscle systems to single-joint, isolation exercises designed to produce fearsome adaptations in the tiniest muscle. It's a stark reality that it doesn't really take much to construct a real, results-producing gym that outclasses the contemporary Gold's Gyms, the encroaching Borg-like Planet Fitness, or even the post-modern YMCA in result potential. The devil, however, is in the details.

Bringing the Gym Home

Beyond the equipment, what we want to do is bring the gym experience home. Not just any gym, but the best parts of every gym you've ever trained in or wanted to train at. Maybe you want to imagine yourself at Gold's Gym in Venice, CA during the golden age of bodybuilding in the 1970s—the place where Arnold, Franco, Frank and Dave trained. On the other hand, you might want to go completely hardcore and emulate the dungeon-like atmosphere of Temple Gym in Birmingham, England, where Dorian Yates forged his muscles under the illumination of a few light bulbs. The point is, you decide and move forward with that overall theme. So, we need to concern ourselves with both the stage and the equipment in order to pull off a great show.

It's Your Gym—How to Get Started

We'll use a three-step overall strategy to build a great home-based training facility:

1. Select and prepare the location.

2. Obtain baseline equipment.

3. Enhance the experience.

Much of the rest of this book describes this process in detail, starting with the first and often most important decision you need to make.

③

Location, Location, Location

From the onset, Ray Kroc, the progenitor of McDonald's, realized the importance of location to his success in selling hamburgers. Similarly, the decision regarding the location of your home gym will become a determinant factor in your ultimate success as a bodybuilder. Where you decide to put your gym is just as important as what you put in it—maybe more so. Let's see why.

The variety, effectiveness and safety of a bodybuilding gym requires three key architectural items—a solid, level foundation (the floor), adequate size and an appropriate ceiling height. Combined, these aspects will largely determine the success of your eventual location.

The Floor

Squats and presses demand a level, solid floor for safety and effectiveness. Every other movement likes this as well. Sure, we've seen the pictures and read the stories about our troops stationed in Iraq or Afghanistan using makeshift lifting equipment, standing in dirt or sand. In fact, much of the third world that lifts (and they do), often lifts in the same substandard conditions and they do get results. But what we are looking for is an environment conducive to optimal results—a level, solid floor, preferably on the ground floor, constructed of cement, or at the least, thick, heavy wood in order to provide safety first, and an unforgiving base for effort. That's why basements and garages do so well for home gyms.

The critical factor here is one of simple physics—force transfer—we don't want any of the force transferred into the floor (or your shoes—I'll discuss that later)—and that's what happens with less than solid surfaces, such as sand, dirt, gravel and thin wood. Existing wood floors can be reinforced with additional wood, such as ¾" plywood, so that's always an alternative if the basement or garage is not available. Placing wood reinforcement on top of an existing, unstable structure (carpet) is not a viable safe option when dealing with progressively heavier loads. In fact, if the underlying floor is not cement (such as a spare room, shed, covered porch, etc.) I strongly suggest laying down sheets of ¾" plywood right from the start to reinforce and protect the underlying floor. There is a reason that powerlifters use a lifting platform. So now you know.

For those wondering if fully loaded racks may strain the load-bearing capabilities of your floor, you can stop worrying. Think about the amount of weight your floors already support. Beds, furniture and people quickly add up to over a thousand pounds. Some fish tanks filled with water can weigh over 500 pounds. Because you won't be putting your rack in the middle of the room, the load will be placed near a wall where the structural engineering of floors is greatest.

One additional note here. If your concrete floor is uneven, try applying self-leveling concrete to correct this issue. It's a cheap fix (about $30-$40) and may save you from injury.

The takeaway lesson here, if you haven't already learned it, is to follow the parable of the wise and foolish builders. Be wise and build your gym upon the rock—not foolish by building it on the sand. Everything flows from this.

Room Size

You don't need a lot of space for a home gym. At minimum, at ten foot square room will work. Because Olympic barbells are seven foot in length, racks are not as wide as bars, and you need to load the bars with plates, this becomes a rote math exercise. A room at ten feet in width allows 1.5 feet of loading space per side and horizontal bar play when in movement. This is the minimal safe environment for handling bars and plates. A one hundred square foot room also allows us just enough space for the baseline equipment I'll discuss below. Because space if often our most limiting dimension in the home gym, this book shows you how to use it wisely.

Ceiling Height

High ceilings are one of the holy grails of a home gym.

Racks and standing presses demand adequate ceiling height. In fact, anything that extends over your head, including extensions for your triceps, jumping rope for conditioning, and step-ups will require something higher than the standard eight foot ceiling height in most homes. If you're lucky or well-off you may have nine foot ceilings in a master bedroom (how's that for intimacy? Honey, let's use the power rack tonight) or all the rooms. Hooray! You're all set. Otherwise, that garage starts looking even more inviting with its nine-foot ceiling. If nine feet is out of reach and out of the question, then your toolbox of exercises becomes more limited. Presses will need to be performed seated. You won't be jumping rope and step-ups will have to step-off. In addition, you'll need to be extra diligent when purchasing a rack, so that its height will fit your ceiling's limitation. But racks that fit within an eight-foot ceiling structure are plentiful.

Because we aren't Olympic lifters or Crossfitters, lack of a nine-foot ceiling is not a deal breaker. So, don't sweat this one too much—just keep the ceiling height in the thought process of selecting a gym location.

Bonus Item: A Door

Doors are underrated. The mere existence of a door assumes an environment physically and mentally separated from the rest of the universe. As Kevin Costner so adeptly illustrated in the baseball movie, *For the Love of the Game*, successful effort is often about "clearing the machine"—working with a clear head, free of distraction. Let's hear it for the door.

Super Bonus Item: A Garage Door

If doors are good, garage doors can be great.

In the 1940s, the fusion of sunshine and cast iron at Muscle Beach showed the world how invigorating it could be to work out in nature's gym. Later, the Russian town of Lyubertsi famously followed suit in the 1980s. Many of us, who have lugged the bench, bar and plates outside in the summer, can attest to this. It's how teen boys used to spend much of their summer, between games of Wiffle™ ball, peeking looks at the older girls sunbathing in their bikinis, riding bikes and swimming (how's that for cross-training). Garage gyms allow a glimpse into that earlier era, more so than any room's open window or big-box gym can offer. On the other end of this spectrum, basement gyms seem so distant, cold and withdrawn, much like the dwarves toiling in Tolkien's mines of Moria.

Garage doors are also the great opportunity cost. For much of the year, they allow you to train in a semi-open environment, with fresh air, cool breezes and sunlight. Remove a wall—get invigorated all over again. Getting the equipment into the garage is a snap. However, when old man winter arrives, that same door offers the barest of protection from the plummeting temperature. Wind has a way of finding you. But hey, that's what sweatshirts and bulking season is for, right?

Speaking of heat and cold, what about electricity?

Electricity

Sure, it should feel exhilarating and electric when you enter your home gym, but that's not what I'm referring to here.

You'll need sufficient access to electrical outlets and wattage if you want things like fans, music, additional lighting or air conditioning. (Don't neglect to check the total wattage available—I discovered that I couldn't run my garage gym's A/C , fan and the pool pump out back at the same time, because they were all on the same garage circuit.) Many of the typical locations for home gyms I'll talk about don't necessarily have central A/C, such as garages, sheds, and older homes. Pay attention to the location of the outlets and your total amps available on the electrical circuit associated with your gym's location.

• • • •

At this point, you should know your location options. You'll need one of the following:

- Garage or portion of the garage
- Basement
- Spare room
- Shed
- Covered porch

Let's see how each stacks up against our three key architectural aspects—floor, ceiling height and overall size. Additionally, we need to start considering some other modern amenities, such as electricity.

Garage

Starting something in your garage has taken on an almost mythical aura over the past century. Amazon, Apple, Harley Davidson, and Disney started life in a garage. While e-commerce, personal computers, motorcycles and damn good entertainment are lofty aspirations, ours is no less humble—to transform ourselves, in the physical sense initially, and like so many others, come out the other end a changed person.

World-renowned strength coach Marty Gallagher writes about his garage gym in his book, *The Purposeful Primitive*:

"My home gym [is] in the unheated garage out back of my country home in South Central Pennsylvania. Our coldest training session was conducted in 19 degree weather and our summer warmest was 102 degrees. The power rack...is the heart and soul of my gym. I have barbells, dumbbells, a few benches, and a single pulley device used for pushdowns and pulldowns (our one machine). Many a World Champion has trained here and the sessions are manic and intense."

Garages and basements are the best locations for a home gym, because they pass muster for floor, ceiling height and size. Most likely, you are starting with a solid concrete floor, which doesn't require any reinforcement before you even pick up a weight. In addition, these locations are tucked away from the main part of the home, helping to nullify noise and providing a clear mental break between work and play. Once past the beginner stages of training, mental focus really becomes the largest dimension in bodybuilding achievement, so let's assist in that area right from the start.

The big downside to garage gyms are the lack of environmental control (it gets either real hot or real cold—or both—sometime during the year). But we can mitigate this to some degree as I'll show you.

Typically, you have two options here—have a garage with a gym in it—this works best with two-car garages, or a gym occupying the entire shell of a former garage. The first option, the one I opted for, allows you to maintain a portion of your existing garage for a vehicle, storage and other miscellaneous use, such as a workbench, tools, etc. When you enter this type of garage, one side is your run of the mill garage, while the other side screams "gym". The second option dedicates the entire garage to exclusive gym use. If you live alone, that's your call. My wife and practicality insisted on the first option. That gave me a 12'x20' space from which to work—luxurious panoply for a powerlifter, and just enough for a couple battle-tested bodybuilders.

Regardless of which garage option you choose, you will need to organize and store items efficiently in order to keep your garage stuff out of your gym. I went from a two-car garage, which housed two cars, five bicycles, two large upright storage cabinets, a workbench, two large wheeled toolboxes, a scrap wood pile, hand truck, two ladders, a snow blower, various sporting goods equipment and kids toys to a single car garage and a gym with all that "stuff" organized efficiently on the car side. It can be done.

The first step was to throw some things out, give others to charity and have a garage sale—, which helped to finance some of my gym equipment purchases. The second car had a new life sitting in the driveway, but the rest of the "stuff" I described found a new home relocated to the "other" side of the garage via strategically rearranging the placement of the cabinets, toolboxes, and woodpile. This second step, of storage and reorganization, allowed the bikes and ladders to be stored vertically via wall hooks, and a couple bike storage systems using cables. When organizing the "garage" side of your garage, use the wall space and ceiling to maximum effect. Home improvement centers sell a large variety of hooks, hanging storage systems and wall-mount shelves for just this purpose. If you've got a lot of scrap wood taking up space, think about how you can repurpose that into some DIY storage solutions. Use the commercial options and the Internet (search for "garage storage" or "garage organization") for inspiration here.

This general procedure of elimination and reorganization works just as well for basement and spare room setups.

Basement

I'm not a fan of basements. They remind me of darkness, dampness and isolation. However, they typically offer plenty of unimpeded room (after elimination and reorganization), good environmental control, easy access to outlets, a door to the upstairs and cement floors, so home gyms often find their natural birth here.

Unless you have a finished basement, this is probably your easiest option. Basements provide the floor and size requirements. Ceiling height may present an issue for racks and standing presses, unless you have nine-foot ceilings.

If your basement is completely finished, what you have is a spare room situation.

Spare Room

Spare rooms are always a good thing. Typically, you probably don't have any "spare" rooms, but maybe one that you can spare—for the required lifting space. Again, elimination and reorganization are big helps here and after some effort, you may find yourself with an open 10'x10' area and a door.

Here, as in the basement, pay attention to ceiling height. Those twelve inches make an awful lot of difference. Ask anybody.

Shed, Carport or Other Structure

All of these offer the possibility of FRESH AIR!

But alas, they also present some unique challenges.

Sheds need to have adequate size (most do), ceiling height (most don't) and a solid floor (may or may not need reinforcing).

A carport or covered porch is our last alternative—and I mean last. If all you've got for gym space is a covered deck, carport, back porch or patio, then it'll be you and the elements. You shouldn't have a problem with the floor (if it's concrete, you're good; otherwise, reinforce it with ¾" plywood, preferably coated with outdoor stain protection), ceiling height or size. It's climate control you will need to deal with.

Sheds, carports, porches, patios and decks are not ideal, but hey, if a man on a remote island in Alaska can train in a shed for thirty years (30!) and produce world-class results, you can certainly improve, no matter the location.

A final thought about location. Throughout the remainder of this book, consider the amount of alteration or permanence you are creating. People move. You may be renting. Families expand and contract. These things limit (or expand) how much you can or want to alter the location for your gym. As you'll see, the way I built and equipped my garage gym allows me to convert it back into a garage for an automobile with minimal effort, if that need arises. Heed the story of the fool, and don't build a boat in the basement and not be able to get it out the door. A little foresight can go a long way here.

• • • •

Regardless of your home gym's eventual location, being at home realizes additional muscle building advantages, particularly with performance nutrition. Your kitchen is right there, so pre- and post-training nutrition becomes effortless and immediate. After taking a quick shower, you can actually have a real meal of solid food (in addition to your quick-acting whey) a couple minutes after your workout, instead of driving home. Things like this provide tiny, incremental optimizations to the overall transformation process. Don't discount it.

Now, once you've decided on the location for your home gym, before you put in any equipment, you need to take a moment and think about the overall layout. Planning the layout will allow you to maximize the space you have for things like—training efficiently, effectively and safely.

Bodybuilding at Home

4

Planning the Layout

It always wise to plan before acting. You know, ready, aim, fire. Firing before aiming is always less likely to produce the results you want. Don't dump your workout gear in a room like you bag your groceries at the checkout.

The key to the layout of your home gym is to plan and execute versatility and efficiency. When planning the layout, sketch it on paper (graph paper really helps), draw it on a whiteboard or tape it out on the floor.

For the sake of this discussion, let's assume our minimal 10'x10' room. Larger rooms will obviously have more space, but the logic of our planning still holds.

First, think of your space as divided into three zones. This logical breakdown helps to frame both the planning process and your eventual workouts.

```
┌─────────────────────────────────────────┐
│                                          │
│               Zone 1                     │
│        Power Rack, Barbell, Bench        │
│                                          │
└─────────────────────────────────────────┘

┌──────────────────────────┐  ┌───────────────┐
│                          │  │               │
│                          │  │    Zone 2     │
│                          │  │   Dumbbells   │
│        Zone 3            │  │       &       │
│ Open floor performance   │  │   Accessory   │
│         area             │  │   Equipment   │
│                          │  │               │
└──────────────────────────┘  └───────────────┘
```

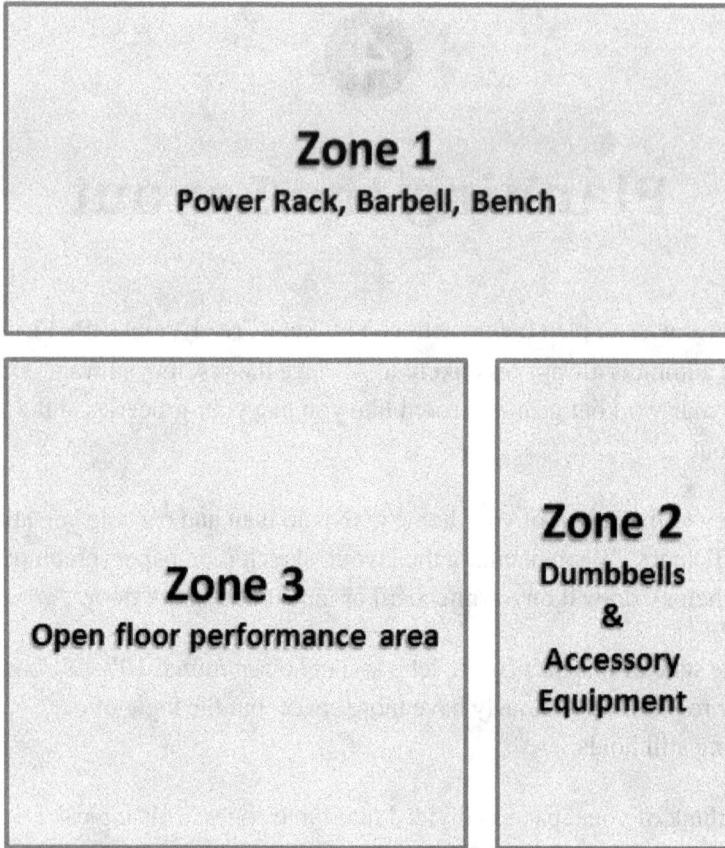

Zone 1: The Heavy Stuff

Your rack will live in Zone 1 and occupy half the room. The barbell and bench can live in the rack most of the time and you should be spending about half of your workout there as well.

Zone 2: Storage

Zone 2 is against one of the other walls. This is where you'll store your dumbbells, bars and accessory equipment. This is also where you'll want to eventually get this stuff up off the floor into some type of vertical storage solutions. I'll discuss your options here as we go along.

Zone 3: Room for Activities

Zone 3 is the remaining open floor area where you'll perform your dumbbell exercises, deadlifts, standing presses and/or cardio. While powerlifters spend the majority of their time in the cage, bodybuilding training often thrives in the open floor area. Expect to spend about half your workout in Zone 3.

This is a simple plan, but it always works, regardless of your location or available space, so don't discount it.

Speaking of discounts, I need to talk about how I'm going to categorize the things you put into your gym, based on the amount of money you have in your wallet.

⑤

Budget, Economy & Luxury

Everyone has a different amount of money they can afford to spend to outfit a home gym. Throughout this book, as I lay out gym components, considerations and options, I want to make sure there is an economically viable option available to everyone, regardless of budget. Think back to my uncle Ray and the Yukon Hercules. My uncle was not a rich man in the monetary sense, often needing to make some of his own equipment in order to produce results. Dennis Weiss endured decades in Spartan conditions with minimal equipment and still thrived in the transformational sense.

Therefore, based on the varying budgets that each of us has to deal with, I categorize most of the items I recommend you add to your home gym into three spending levels: Budget, Economy and Luxury.

Budget

Budget items are just that—the minimal amount you can spend, while still satisfying our goals of safety, reliability and functionality. Items here get you started quickly with little expense. However, even at this budget level, I won't steer you into an option that could hurt you or sacrifice results. These are the items you may have to start with, eventually upgrading to economy alternatives as your resources allow. This is Uncle Ray and Yukon Hercules. Look how far they went.

Note that some budget items are pure gold and have no functional improvement at the economy or luxury level.

Many people get started at the budget level by allocating a monthly home gym 'allowance', based on what they have spent on monthly dues at the local gym. Over time, this trickle approach eventually stocks an excellent home gym in a year or two—one that lasts forever, with no additional expense.

Economy

Think of economy items as a step up from the budget level. Typically, items here are more durable, useful and efficient. These are the items that most of us can afford and are likely to purchase. You'll spend most of your time finding deals on these items.

Luxury

Luxury items are nice to have, but are not a critical component for our bodybuilding purposes. They may make your gym life easier though, as well as providing even more options in the transformational process. If you have the means, buying items in this category can make your home gym legendary.

• • • •

One final note here. The prices and price ranges I list throughout for Budget, Economy and Luxury items were current at the time of writing. Prices change—in modern society they go up (surprise!). What you should direct your attention to is relative prices—for example, note that a budget barbell is about one-half to one-third the cost of an economy bar, or that rubber hex dumbbells run about 150% of the cost per pound of their cast iron brothers. These price relationships hardly ever change.

❻

Setting the Stage

There is more to creating a home gym than just placing workout equipment in a room. The key to establishing an environment ripe for transforming your body –one that enforces constant motivation and self-discipline—is largely environmental and sensory. The mental aspect of training is often far more important than any physical element. You need to program and appease the mind to keep the body invigorated. Flooring, lighting, mirrors, temperature, sound, video and imagery combine in a synergy to keep you wanting to be in that room. Hey, you like the kitchen and living room, right? Therefore, we need to set up the gym to offer similar sensory enticement. Failure to accomplish this just makes working out harder than it has to be—and your local gym already does a good job at that.

Creating the Proper Lifting Environment

Your "proper" lifting environment is highly personal, but shares a few common traits that we need to establish, primarily for safety and effectiveness.

In this section, we'll talk about flooring, lighting, mirrors, how to control the temperature, sound and video systems, visual appeal and a few miscellaneous items that can help make your workouts even more effective.

Flooring

Some type of rubberized flooring is essential for any home gym to protect the floors (whether wood or cement), absorb sweat, allow for easy cleanup, reduce noise (especially important for apartment dwellers) and maybe most importantly protect you and your joints. Regardless of your desire or determination, you will drop weights. Grip slips, training to failure, and incorrect setups can quickly—and I mean quickly—sidestep even the best-laid intentions. So plan in advance and get some rubber flooring. But not just any rubber flooring.

Rubber Flooring Considerations

Flooring should be simple, right? Well, it is if you know what parameters you need to consider, their effects and the effect on your wallet. Let's see what's involved.

Underlying Base

If you are starting on a cement floor, then proceed ahead to the remainder of this discussion. Otherwise, for you carpet-based or wood floor participants, I highly suggest putting down at least one (and preferably two) layer of three quarter-inch plywood. This will create a solid base for the rubber floor that goes on top and will provide additional protection if heavy weights are dropped during deadlifts.

Density

This is the most important aspect in flooring. For weight training activities, we want a flooring material that is extremely dense, providing almost zero give (this isn't floor aerobics), allowing us to transfer minimal force into the floor and maximal force into our efforts. Note that flooring density is not something directly specified on most floor products—look for descriptions that include the words "softness", "running", "bounding" or "jumping". We won't be doing much of that, so avoid those. Finally, be aware that most small, 2'x2' interlocking "gym" flooring sold in packages does not have the required density to match our weight training requirements or provide the necessary stability to support things like power racks. These mass-market interlocking rubber tiles are fine for placing under a piece of cardio equipment or anything that doesn't move around and will still protect your floor.

Thickness

Gym flooring is available in various advertised thicknesses, from ¼" to
¾". Keep in mind that thickness drives price, so the thicker flooring we
desire is also more expensive. Couple the flooring's density with thickness
to determine which flooring will work for you—denser flooring can
mitigate some amount of thickness.

Durability

Primarily, thickness and density determine durability. Dense, thick
flooring tends to last a lot longer, so look for that, especially flooring that
advertises durability to "dropped weights".

Interlocking, Rolls, or Mats

Regardless of the available space, you are not going to be able to just plop
one giant piece of flooring down and be done with it. Your gym floor must
be pieced together—whether it is multiple mats abutting or interlocked
with each other, or sheets of flooring cut from a roll. Interlocking flooring
increases the cost significantly due to increased manufacturing processes,
but allows for the easiest installation. With mats, you'll need to place them
securely up against each other and may need to cut them to fit your space.
If cutting is required, be aware that thickness and density determines your
ease of cutting. Most mats can be cut with a utility knife, but some thick,
dense mats will either provide you with a vigorous grip and forearm
workout or you'll need an electric saw.

Stability & Fit

When assembling your gym floor from mats or from a roll, you want to
ensure that everything fits together securely and stays that way. With
interlocking mats, this is a non-issue. Rolls and individual mats may
require some adhesive under them to keep them in place. Even with heavy,
thousand pound racks with plates, I've still seen rubber flooring separate
from each other over time. Typically, this happens with smooth underlying
surfaces, such as plywood, coated/sealed garage or basement floors and
even hardwood floors. If this happens to you, your local hardware or carpet

store sells inexpensive adhesive strips for securing the mats at the corner edges.

Color

To some this may seem a minor characteristic—just pick black and get on with it—but to others, aesthetics provide inspiration. Commercial flooring offers the most options here. In gym flooring black dominates, with various shades of gray following. Tan, blue, and even shades of yellow are available as well. Additionally, some manufacturers sell various speckled designs over the base color. Speckled flooring tends to obscure minor dirt particles or stains.

Cost

As I mentioned earlier, flooring density and thickness are the prime cost drivers. In this case, you really do get what you pay for. Because we require dense, thick floors for our efforts, plan to spend about $2/square foot to properly cover the floor of your home gym. And that leads us to the big question here…

How Much Flooring Do I Need?

The answer—everywhere you plan on handling a loaded weight. Going back to that 3-Zone layout, that means you need the flooring under your rack (Zone 1) and under your bench and feet (Zone 3). Whether you put any in Zone 2 (storage) may be determined by both your budget and by how much pain you can tolerate if something heavy does get dropped there. I do know that in my case, dropping a 100lb dumbbell off the rack and cracking the underlying floor would give my wife ample reason to send me to Zone 4 (The Doghouse), at least temporarily.

Based on all of the parameters listed above, you should strongly consider two types of flooring—commercial rollout flooring and horse stall mats.

Horse Stall Mats

When I suggest the use of horse stall mats for home gym flooring, sometimes I get the question, "Do these things hold up?" Well, most horses are relatively heavy, averaging 1100lbs. Most farmers I know don't buy stuff that wears out quickly. So yeah, they hold up. That fact that they are black, ¾" thick, weigh about 100lbs apiece, don't move when placed, usually include a 10-year warranty, and are affordable (about $40 for a 4'x6' mat—that's $1.50-$1.75/square foot) for the quality makes them even more appealing for us. Stall mats are also relatively easy to cut (using box cutters) to fit your exact space requirements or to cut holes for anchoring power racks, if necessary. Be aware that these things are heavy (100lbs for a 4'x6' mat), so shipping them to you is probably going to be out of the question. You'll need a pickup truck, minivan or a car with a hatch or large trunk to transport these from a farm supply store—and you'll get a nice workout in the process!

For my home gym, I used ten horse stall mats to cover my 12'x20' foot area. I did have to use small adhesive stickers to hold the mats securely in place and tightly against each other—even with hundreds of pounds of plates and dumbbells sitting on top of them—because my garage floor was finished with a smooth protective, yet slippery, coating.

Commercial Rollout Flooring

Most commercial gyms use seamless rubber flooring in the free weight and exercise machine areas. This flooring is relatively durable and looks great, but comes at a steeper cost. Commercial rollout gym flooring is available in various widths (32", 36", 42" and 48") and just about any color, pattern, thickness (from ¼" to ¾"), and type (interlocking, mats, rollout). When you avoid the thinner variety (1/4" thickness), you encounter your biggest obstacle here—cost. This stuff can quickly get prohibitively expensive. You'll see typical prices quoted by the square foot, from an absolute low of $2, the more common $3, upwards to, "Call for price". If "Call for price" gives you pause, then you're probably already priced out of this category. Here, even a small 10'x10' home gym will set you back somewhere between $200-$300 for the flooring. But it looks and works magnificently.

Check your local home improvement centers first before exploring other dedicated sports retail merchants. This stuff is dense, so you can opt for a minimal thickness of ½". I would advise on getting the widest roll possible, probably the 48" variety. Typically, a 20' minimum roll is required for purchase, so you can opt for a single roll at that length to cover most of our 10'x10' minimal footprint. That will set you back about $200.

Budget Flooring ($80)

Two horse stall mats. That provides 8'x12' coverage—just about enough to completely cover our recommended minimal home gym footprint (10'x10') and more than enough to place under your power rack, bench and dumbbells. They are also the most durable of all the options listed here.

Economy Flooring ($120+)

Enough horse stall mats to cover your entire gym floor area. Because most common horse stall mats are 4'x6' in size at about $40 each, measure your floor and multiply the number of mats you would need by $40 to arrive at your total. For our recommended minimal home gym footprint, you need three of these.

Luxury Flooring ($200+)

Commercial rollout gym flooring. High price per square foot, but looks the best, performs well and requires minimal installation and cutting for fit.

Lighting

While you only require enough lighting in your home gym to ensure that you can put plates on bars, select dumbbells, and not trip over anything, bodybuilders tend to seek enough light to analyze their lifting technique, identify physique imperfections and yes, admire the gains. Guilty as charged.

How much light does a bodybuilder need? That depends on goals and vanity.

If your goal is the competitive stage, at any level, then you want to provide the same level of unforgiving illumination that the stage presents—or at least as close to that as you can simulate. For the narcissists, it's much like the story of Goldilocks and the three bears. You don't want too much light or too little, but just enough to accentuate the display of muscle development and separation, whether perceived or actual. The henchman in this drama is the mirror, of course.

For those outcasts lifting in sheds, electricity is ideal but not required. Battery-powered fluorescent lighting is available relatively cheaply—much cheaper than renting a Ditch-Witch and digging an electrical conduit to your shed.

Lighting Considerations

Based on your goals and vanity, there are several aspects of lighting that you may want to consider.

Size of Room

This is the primary concern. I shouldn't have to say it, but the larger the space you are trying to light, the more lighting you will need, unless shadows are your friend. For our minimal 10x10 foot layout, a single, centralized lighting source in the ceiling will do fine. The type of lighting to have comes next.

Type

This boils down to florescent lighting or not. Florescent is much less forgiving (the truth is bared!) to the physique artist but more closely mimics stage lighting conditions for those with competitive aspirations. The downside is the cost. Simple single bulb lighting is cheaper, quicker to install, replace and dispose. However, it tends to obscure the truth and accentuate the mirage.

Wattage

Why do you need to know the wattage of your lighting? If you are lifting in a spare bedroom, you probably don't need or care about that. But, if you decide to start installing some florescent lighting—especially more than one strip, and you want to run that A/C window unit and the vacuum to clean up the floor from all the chalk and everything suddenly shuts off—you get concerned. Each electrical circuit can only handle a certain amount of load, so do yourself a quick favor and go through the one-time mental exercise of adding up the wattage of everything you will ever use at the same time on that circuit—lights, A/C or heater, vacuum, etc. Either adjust your lighting aspirations from there or be cognizant that you won't be able to perform some of those tasks simultaneously.

There are other minor lighting specs and formalities here, like lumens and color. Stick with white light and forget the lumens, unless your livelihood depends on it.

When I was converting half of my two-car garage into my garage gym (12'x20'), I replaced the single 100-watt light bulb with two banks of 4ft, four-bulb florescent lights. For about $200 I was able to provide more effective lighting than my local Gold's Gym. My workout partners noticed the difference immediately.

Budget Lighting ($0)
I'm almost certain Lincoln lifted by candlelight. For us modern lifters, a single light bulb will do. You probably already have this as your existing lighting.

Economy Lighting ($60)
One fluorescent light panel (2 or 4 bulb—4 recommended) with 4 or 8ft bulbs.

Luxury Lighting ($150-$300)
Multiple 4 bulb fluorescent light panels, using 8ft bulbs. You'll see EVERYTHING, every physical imperfection, every ounce of muscle—and fat. Make sure you can handle the truth or sublet your home gym for minor surgical operations, because it will be lit like an operating room.

Mirrors

If there were no mirrors, there would be no bodybuilders. You'll need to include at least one small mirror in order to monitor your performance, conditioning and progress. We are bodybuilding here, not powerlifting. Let me tell you what I think is "small".

Mirror Considerations

Size

As a bodybuilder, you need to see your entire physique, from head to toe. Therefore, you'll want a full-length mirror, something that is at least four feet in height. Six foot is preferable, especially if you are confined in a small 10'x10' space and do most of your work inside the power rack.

Speaking of the rack, try to install a mirror that is about as wide as the rack. Coupled with a six foot height, this will provide you with ample mirror space right where you need it. (For your powerlifter friends who want to lift with you, just hang a sheet over the mirror when they lift—they'll feel at home.) An quick, inexpensive way to achieve this is to get two closet mirrors and hang them side by side.

Thickness

One problem with cheap, mass-market closet mirrors is the "circus effect". You know what this is. It's when you look at yourself and see a thinner or fatter reflection of yourself.

I remember decades ago when I propped up a cheap cardboard-backed closest mirror against the basement wall and started curling my Weider sand-filled dumbbells. For a minute, I thought I achieved a 20" arm and was on my way to Mr. Olympia.

Hopefully, distortions like this are due to the mirror and not any body dysmorphia condition you may have. In any case, cheap, thin mirrors, especially when mounted only at the edges creates distortion and affects true reflection, which is important to the physique competitor. Thicker mirrors, such as the one in your bathroom, offer a more accurate reflection, along with a heftier price.

Placement

The size, especially the height of the mirror you have will largely dictate its placement, offset from the floor. Taller mirrors can—and should be—mounted lower toward the floor. Make sure you can see your calves and the top of your head in the space you will be working out.

Installation

The only real key to hanging your mirror(s) is to apply some Gorilla Glue to each square foot of the mirror's backing in order to secure the entire mirrors surface to the wall on the same plane. In addition to the mounting hardware, this will go far toward reducing any "circus mirror" effects from a slightly bowed installation. This is how the professionals do it, and it only takes a minute of extra effort, so be wise and follow suit.

One final consideration—the more mirror space you have, the larger the home gym appears. Sometimes illusions can motivate and inspire.

Budget Mirrors ($10)

A cheap single closet door mirror from Wal-Mart (or your favorite mass-market retailer). They are thin and cheap. You may get a circus-like result, making you look either bigger or smaller than you actually are, but it's hard to beat a $10 bill to provide continuous visual feedback and check your form consistently.

Economy Mirrors ($100-$300)

Move up to sliding-door mirrors. These are thicker and wider than the cheap closet mirrors. Home improvement centers sell these (usually in pairs, but ask if they have any damaged units with a single mirror and negotiate). You can get two for about $100 and cover a 6'x6' area right behind your power rack.

Luxury Mirrors ($350+)

These are commercial mirrors found in gyms, hair salons, and ahem, adult entertainment venues. Typically they come in panels that are 6' tall, and range up to eight feet in width. They are thick, and offer true reflections and perspective. This is the option I went with, because, well I'm vain and was raised (and grew) in commercial gyms with these things covering just about all the walls. It provided me with an easy transition to the home gym, because I essentially duplicated that part of the environment I was used to. Sometimes, you can find great deals on these when any of the types of establishments I listed above go out of business or are remodeling. Also, check with commercial glass and mirror business to see if they have any damaged mirrors that they will cut down for you. Other than that, the Internet is your friend here—there are some great deals to be had.

Climate Control

Over the past 25 years, I've trained at several gyms, from a small iron-based gym to the large commercial franchised operations. In each case, there came a time when the climate control became—noticeable. You shouldn't notice the temperature or humidity in a gym. For several years, the running joke among some of the hardcore lifters was to make all your gains in the spring and fall, because you'll be sweating your ass off, gasping for breath in the summer, and freezing to death in the winter. Summer and winter were for maintenance. Strength trainer extraordinaire, Marty Gallagher, may write about the intense training sessions in his garage gym in the heat and height of summer, with the mercury rising upwards of 100 degrees, but Marty is a better man than me at surviving and thriving in that environment. Likewise for the ice-chipping Yukon Hercules.

In his book, *Power: A Scientific Approach*, Fred Hatfield ("Dr. Squat") discusses the 22 factors that affect strength—and strength lies at the heart of all physical activity, including bodybuilding. One of those 22 factors contributing to strength is the environment (heat, cold, humidity, etc.). Additionally, environmental aspects have spillover effects on the psychoneural strength factor of focus/concentration. So, you can see why this might be something to consider for optimal home gym training.

Think about your best workouts. What do you remember about them? I venture it probably isn't the heat or the cold, the humidity or the frost. It was the workout, pure and simple. Climate was not a detrimental characteristic. And that's what we're after here.

The weather outside and your gym's location will dictate your need for temperature control. If your gym is in a spare room in the house with central air and heat, you're all set. Basement and garage dwellers or those in houses without central air may need to add some air conditioning. Others may not see the need, depending on geographical location or fortitude. Similar situations concern heat.

Let's look at the options.

Fans

Fans are a godsend in hot environments. High-speed, commercial fans are even better. Sometimes, the difference between getting that tenth rep on squats and packing it in is a simple blast of air. However, in hot, humid environments, fans only move around the existing air—it isn't really getting any cooler, although your body's cooling system may think it is. And that's why fans work.

The size of your gym and budget will dictate the type of fan you should get. At the low end, you can find cheap fans at yard sales, consignment stores, or Walmart. They will move a minimum to modicum of air in small spaces. High-speed, commercial fans, like those used in warehouses, barns or other large structures are, obviously, more expensive but can move a significant amount of air throughout larger environs. They also tend to be loud, something to consider if you listen to music or talk with your comrades while training.

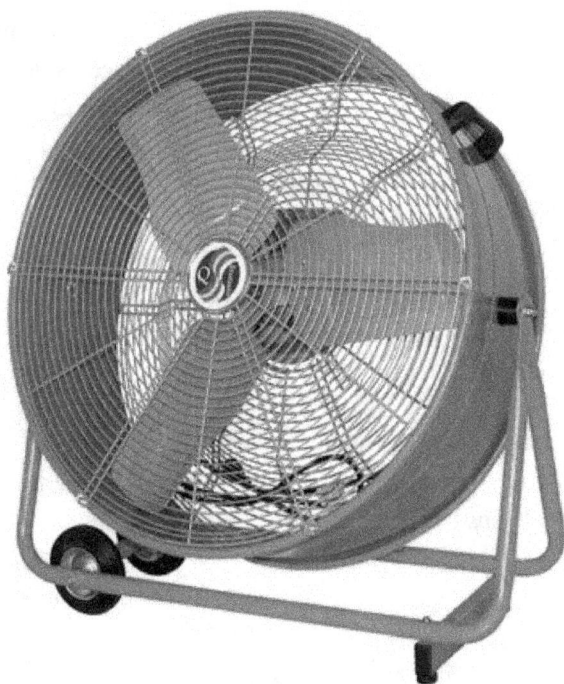

Because July in Maryland gets both really hot and really humid, I opted for an industrial fan that I could set up right next to the rack. In times like these, I can't hear much over the fan, but I sure don't miss a rep or a lift due to the sweltering environment.

Air Conditioning Unit

If a fan doesn't do it for you, move up to an air conditioning unit. If your home gym has a window, you can go for a window-based unit. These are much more efficient than portable A/C units are—however; if you are concerned with the exterior aesthetics of your home, keep in mind that they can present a visual eyesore sticking out of the window. Because my garage has two street-facing windows, my first inclination was to get a window unit. However, because I like to stay happily married, my wife insisted that we not be the only house in our nice neighborhood with an ugly eyesore of a window A/C unit sticking right out there for onlookers to gawk at. Because the punishment from a wife can be quite severe, I opted for a portable unit.

Now, portable A/C units do require some type of outside opening for exhaust to escape, but most come with a window-based exhaust panel (about 6" high) that significantly minimizes any exterior issues.

Whether you opt for a window-based or portable model, make sure you know how many amps the device will consume on your electrical circuit. In my case, I can run the air conditioning, fan and lights in my garage—but turning on the outside light exceeds my circuit's capacity, putting a temporary end to any nighttime training sessions, and necessitating a trip to the breaker box.

The combination of air conditioning and a fan really can't be beat when the dog days of summer arrive. As my younger training partners would attest—it really keeps the "gainz" comin'.

Space Heater

While heat seems to sap my strength like kryptonite, some of my better workouts have come with Jack Frost nipping at my nose. After an appropriate warm-up, I can train in cold environments without any ill effects. However, when my home gym's temperature starts falling below 50 degrees, some heat is a welcome workout companion.

For heating smaller spaces, such as a home gym, a portable space heater is an efficient solution. Now, there are all types of these things, and you can spend a lot of time researching and comparing them, but the ones I find the safest (remember safety!), easiest to use and efficient are the simple electrical forced air models. Just remember to take into account the amps used and you'll have a quick solution to those subterranean temperatures. When my garage gym falls below 50 degrees (a thermometer is a useful addition to the wall), I turn on my space heater.

Finally, if you are lucky enough to be lifting in a garage gym, open the garage door in the spring and fall for some great fresh air, an enlarged training area and some wonderful atmosphere. This is why garage gyms become so valuable—you can have both the original Gold's Gym and the Venice Muscle Beach iron pit at the same time. This is what flocks training partners to your setup.

Don't Forget Insulation

If your home gym will be located in the basement, garage or a shed, don't neglect the importance of insulation. When I bought my home, the garage was unfinished and offered me the opportunity to insulate the walls, ceiling, windows, and garage doors myself. I didn't skimp on the insulation then and it's really paid off now in both summer and winter.

Think about your location. Sheds don't come with insulation. If you lift there, add some. If you lift in an unfinished basement, consider some wall insulation or hang insulated curtains from the ceiling joists. This will reduce the amount of space that your heater needs to handle and keep the heat localized to your setup. I hung a strip of insulated curtains between the car portion of my two-car garage and my gym portion and it's really helped the space heater to drive up the temperature quickly in the dead of winter.

The budget, economy and luxury options below relate to those of you training in sheds, garages and unfinished basements. Otherwise, you're indoors and probably good to go.

Budget Climate Control ($0-$30)
Either tough it out, lift in the house, move to Hawaii, or get a fan. In the winter, layer up and warm-up.

Economy Climate Control ($100-$300)
Get an industrial fan. It'll blow you away.

Luxury Climate Control ($300+)
Get an industrial fan and an air conditioner. Make it like Hawaii. In the coldest of days, turn on the space heater about 30-60 minutes before training begins. Notice nothing and just lift.

Sound, Video & Visual Appearance

When the last commercial gym I trained at first opened, they played country music over the sound system. That was an error in judgment and management, a mismatch to the membership profile and they quickly corrected, shifting to Top 40 tunes. Somehow, slowly over time, that morphed into a bad mix of dance music, hip-hop and rap. To me, it was so bad, it actually became a motivator to get in and out of the gym as quickly as possible. That's my opinion. And that's the general auditory issue and your home gym solution.

Here's where the benefits of the home gym become visually and audibly apparent. You don't have to strap on ear buds and an MP3 player—just crank up your music and let your ears breath.

Don't underestimate the motivational aspects of music and video. Placing yourself into a heightened emotional state via music will permit you to train heavier and harder. Think of it as auditory smelling salts.

Sound & Fury

To this day, when I am lifting and hear Motley Crue's *Dr. Feelgood*, it takes me back to my lifting genesis, along with all the heart and desire of that time. Full power then commences. (For hardcore bodybuilding aficionados, almost nothing compares to the full-volume experience of the soundtrack to *Conan the Barbarian* while training.)

Besides promoting work capacity, quickness of movement and endurance, music can be a big motivational aspect for many—look at the number of folks in gyms wearing those earbuds. Sure, some are avoiding the cookie-cutter, pop-music garbage pumped through the overhead sound system, but many are lifting to their music, and their volume levels. Again, freedom reigns.

For the home gym, audible solutions are easy and varied. If funds are limited, try an old radio (remember those?). For a more modern approach, hook your phone or MP3 player to a speaker system. If you are in an apartment, have neighbors close by, or the kids are sleeping, use a radio/Bluetooth-based headphone. One day, while browsing through the local Goodwill store, I scored an MP3-based speaker system for $10. Only the remote control was missing. Big deal. Now, when my younger training partners come over, we lift to my 80s rock or their grunge metal. Smiles and high-fives abound.

Sometimes you want to give the ears a break and use a video for motivation.

Video Stimulation

I find it useful for both instructional and motivational purposes to have some type of video device in my home gym. The Internet is ripe with high-quality instructional training videos, seminars and workouts, specific to your needs. The trick is sifting through the morass to get to the truly valuable stuff. Even a simple analog television hooked up to a VHS or DVD player offers ample alternatives and cheap options. Add a wall-mounted (save the floor space), Internet-connected SmartTV (or bring your tablet) to your gym for the ultimate horizon of options, opening the world of personal training, free daily workouts, unlimited inspiration and streaming of almost inexhaustible content, many from the masters themselves. Take advantage of the impending fact that today's relatively 'new' SmartTVs are the standard TV of tomorrow. At some point, all those 'simple' flat-screen TVs will be sold at bargain-basement prices. That's when you make your move.

I was able to purchase a SmartTV on sale in January (that's the best time of year for deals on new televisions) that I mounted above my garage gym mirrors. The TV includes a USB port, so I went out and bought an inexpensive USB memory stick, visited YouTube and downloaded dozens of hours of training videos to the stick. Insert the stick into the TV and instant virtual gym, complete with all the sights and sounds of the commercial landscape. Now, my wife was able to learn kettlebell training, yoga and have access to ready-made, paced dumbbell training workouts. Her enthusiasm and results reflected this expanded training universe and we both ended up winning.

Often, just turning on the TV for background 'white noise' can transform a solidary home gym into an illusory place full of people. Mind tricks like this can have huge impacts on training results over the long-term.

A final word of caution here—beware the distraction of television, the Internet, YouTube or any other streaming video. Any video you pump into your home gym is for motivational purposes—it should not distract you from training. If it does, turn it off or get rid of it. That was the premise for legendary trainer Vince Gironda's rule—he didn't allow any music to be played in his Studio City, CA gym. Just lift—and get out.

Visual Appeal

Regardless of your audio and video options, enhancing the overall visual appeal of your home gym is another step in calling you to this place. That's what we want.

If you can, consider painting the walls, or at least, painting some color highlights. Hang some posters. Flags are a staple of many basement and garage gyms. Much like an Olympian training in Colorado Springs, some individuals like to channel this and hang the American flag in their gym. Others prefer Iron Maiden posters. Whatever gets you motivated, hang it, display it and feed off it.

Try posting some before and after pictures on your wall this time, instead of the Internet. Find some pictures of your goal physique (be reasonable here) or photos of your old training partners. The options here are really limitless.

Budget Audio/Visual ($0-$50)
A radio and an old TV/VCR/DVD. If you don't have these offhand, yard sales reign supreme. I bet you can find a copy of *Pumping Iron* on VHS for a couple bucks.

Economy Audio/Visual ($150-$200)
Use a tablet or mount a small flat-screen TV on the wall and connect your MP3 player to a speaker dock.

Luxury Audio/Visual ($300+)
Get some surround-sound Bluetooth speakers and a SmartTV. Congratulations, you've just elevated your simple home gym to world-class levels of inspiration, education and envy. This level of audio and video is typically enough to draw in training partners. Make sure the training matches the environment.

Miscellaneous Items

While radios, TVs, flags and posters are nice to have in a home gym, they aren't essential. A couple items do have practical use and are inexpensive.

Clock

Every home gym should have a clock. Time is an essential element of any type of training, and bodybuilding is no exception. Besides the typical between set rest intervals of 1-2 minutes, hypertrophy-based training—especially at the intermediate and advanced levels—includes many time-based intensity-boosting techniques. A clock that allows you to see the seconds elapsing is essential for executing these techniques with precision.

This is also where it's good to go old school and have a large clock with a clear, sweeping second hand, like the kind you used to stare at in school, waiting for the class to end, except now you'll be watching and waiting for the next set to start or lactic acid to dissipate.

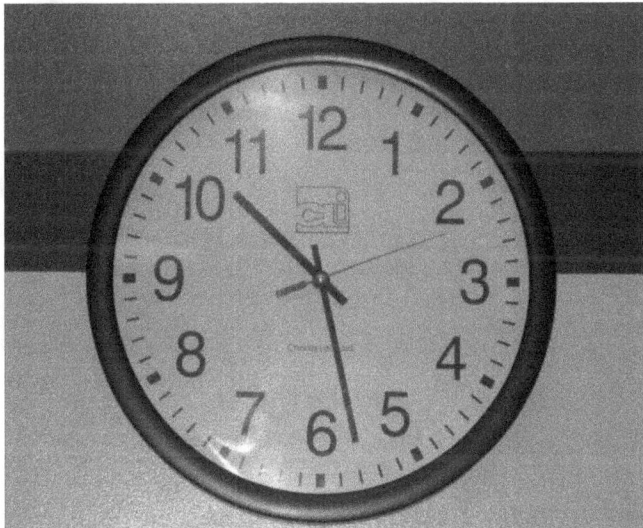

If you don't already have a spare clock lying around, you should be able to pick one up with a second hand for $5-$20. I like the ones with the red second hand. Clear, bold and ominous.

Dry Erase Board (Whiteboard) or Chalkboard

In my home gym, I attached a small 11"x14" whiteboard to the wall that I picked up from a local office supply store for about $20. This is where I write the monthly workouts that my kids follow.

Besides writing out workouts, these things are great for writing goals, accomplishments and motivational quotes—"Stop saying, 'I Wish' and start saying 'I Will'", "Confront Your Fear", "Get to Living or Get to Dying", "You Can't Find Arnold in a Bottle", "This is Where Champions Train", etc. It's also good for immediately communicating to training partners what's about to go down, as soon as they step foot in the place.

I suggest getting the biggest chalkboard or whiteboard you can fit in your gym. That will give you plenty of room to write goals, workouts, motivational and inspirational quotes and your accomplishments—all at the same time. Final tip—use a camera to take occasional pictures of what's on your board. You probably won't realize the importance of that information until after you erase it.

Hooks

As you acquire various pieces of accessory equipment (I'll get to this stuff later), it's helpful to get some stick-on wall hooks at your local home improvement store in order to hang things like a lifting belt, dip belt and jump rope. This gets them off the floor and gives you more room to train and not trip over something. Get them as you need them.

• • • •

In this section, I hoped you've seen that after setting the stage, your home gym should be a place you want to spend time, not somewhere you have to force yourself to go. Attention to detail is important here, because it comes down to the little things that can keep the training fire burning long into life. This attention to detail extends from the location setup into every aspect of the gym equipment you acquire.

7

The Equipment

Legendary bodybuilder and three-time Mr. Universe Reg Park, started his bodybuilding career in the 1940s in a wooden-floored spare room with a pair of dumbbells, a barbell and some plates.

Free weights—barbells, dumbbells and plates—form our core equipment and training strategy. They are by far the best apparatus ever designed to get in shape, lose body fat, build muscle, increase strength and fix almost every possible ailment. Training with free weights causes your entire system to adapt and change. Yes, your muscles get stronger, but so do your bones, tendons, ligaments, heart, vessels, lungs—everything. Consistent application of weight-bearing exercise has proven to reduce later-life incidence of arthritis, heart disease, diabetes, bone loss, and age-related injuries. Noted strength coach Mark Rippetoe has consistently preached that strong people are harder to kill and generally live longer. It's a stark, but true reality. Another reality is that in today's glamorized product world, about the only things that never wear out are an anvil and a classic frying pan—both constructed from cast iron. We're in luck.

While commercial gyms spend the majority of their budget on fancy cardio devices with built-in screens and fans, and powder-coated, padded exercise machines, the most effective and inexpensive equipment they have—the barbells and dumbbells—barely show up on the budget and get surprisingly light use (until you realize that humans prefer easier things to harder things). We'll use this reality with our goal of effective maximization of results, given your budget and space, to deliver a general equipment strategy that maximizes your results, health and longevity.

Think about the equipment you've used at gyms. What did you like and not like? Use that knowledge to eliminate the typical gap between home and commercial gym equipment. In fact, use that knowledge to *exceed* the commercial gym. That's the key here.

Here's a simple example.

At my local Gold's Gym, I can choose from three E-Z Curl bars if I want to use that bar for curls. However, I really like bars with heavy knurling—and at my gym I have none like that. So I satisfice and use what is provided. Not at home. I was able to find a heavily knurled Olympic E-Z Curl bar at Play It Again Sports for $20. No more satisficing and on to my next gap to close.

You shrink the gap by raising the bar. Commercial gyms have fixed chinning bars. Mine are adjustable in width and grip setting. Commercial gyms dumbbell sets ascend in 5lb increments. Mine ascend in 2.5lb increments. (I'll show you why that's important later.) You get the point.

The purpose of all the equipment is to learn, master and progressively overload the five fundamental human movements, as Dan John so eloquently stresses (the push, pull, hinge, squat and carry)—this is our base. From there, we need equipment that facilitates overload of single-joint movements, so central to bodybuilding success.

Our first goal is to obtain the minimum amount of equipment necessary to start with and expand in a logical progression from there. I'll show you how to do that. By no means, do you need or should you fully equip your home gym from the onset. Building the perfect home gym that fits your needs should take a while and grow as your strength and development grows. It will be much more manageable on your wallet as well.

In this section, I'll give you the who, what, why, when, where and how of the tools of our trade, so that you can make the best decision for yourself regarding your equipment.

I'll use the following formula with each item:

First, I'll give you a description and photo of the item I'm talking about, followed by why it's important—or not necessary. This categorizes each piece of equipment as **Essential, Recommended, or Optional**. The discussion includes various advantages and disadvantages regarding the general piece of equipment itself, as well as specific nuances to be aware of. Following is a summary and discussion of things to consider with this piece of equipment, finishing up with tips on where to purchase (new, used or DIY) and recommendations regarding specific manufacturers. Finally, I'll provide a list of exercises that each particular piece of equipment opens up to you.

I'm presenting the equipment in optimal order of acquisition. Acquire the first items first, followed by the subsequent equipment. Don't worry if you already have some of the stuff mentioned later on—I'll show you how to incorporate or eliminate all of these items.

General Equipment Strategy

I suggest following some basic rules when deciding which equipment to purchase (whether new or used) or to build.

Make Smart Investments

Don't buy or build things you don't need. Do buy or build things that can serve general or multi-purpose use. Buy or build things that will last. One of the main purposes of this book is to guide you toward these smart investments. Read on.

Make Timely Investments

The old adage 'timing is everything' holds true for your equipment purchases as well. Many big box sporting goods and department stores discount fitness equipment just as you are shoving that third helping of turkey and stuffing into your mouth at Thanksgiving. Similarly, look for heavy discounts and clearance sales on fitness equipment just as the groundhog is ceremoniously yanked from his hole at the beginning of February. Spring is sprung and all those New Year's resolutions are already dying on the vine—or at Gold's Gym—so retailers need to clear space for shorts, swimming trunks and more yoga mats.

Prioritize your purchases

Remember one of the primary differences between bodybuilders and powerlifters—bodybuilders need to acquire a greater diversity of movement mastery than powerlifters. So, while every general strength athlete and powerlifter should start with a bar, a bench and some plates, the novice bodybuilder, especially with a limited budget, can get much further down that road of movement patterns by taking a slightly different starting tactic.

If you want the greatest exercise diversity and quickest results as you slowly accumulate your equipment, you should use the following strategy for prioritizing your purchases:

1. Dumbbells

2. Adjustable Bench

3. Barbell

4. Plates

5. Rack

6. Pulley/Cable System

7. Additional bars

8. Accessory Equipment

I'll explain the logic in this ordering in more detail below.

One thing to note—if you already have some of the stuff listed above, start filling in your equipment gaps from the top of the list down. And if you stumble across a great deal on something regardless of it's ordering on the list, get it. Worry about how it fits into the priority order later. Great deals are great because they are uncommon. Take advantage—remember, this is a long-term endeavor.

Quality Matters

Home gym equipment needs to be of high quality for primarily for safety and secondarily for durability. Buy the best you can afford—it will last you forever and not send you to the emergency room.

Lawnmowers and mixing bowls offer good examples of this.

Years ago, I was like Mr. Suburban and purchased a riding lawnmower from a home improvement store. Now I could cut my one-acre lawn in about an hour with the mower's 46" deck. It wasn't the fastest mower around, but it got the job done. Then, a couple years later, things started to break. The walk to the shed became a dreaded event, wondering what would break this time. Eventually, I decided to sell the mower and get a used commercial zero-turn mowing beast—for the same price I paid for the new mower. Except this one had a 60" deck, mowed at three times the speed and was clearly constructed of materials meant to withstand abuse. That first year, I gained an additional three days of my life back, not to mention peace of mind. Think about this when purchasing a power rack.

Most people like a nice set of color-coordinated mixing bowls. Others just buy any mixing bowl that will let you mix things in it. Then they break, one gets lost or left at a party somewhere, or your color scheme changes. I threw all of our mixing bowls away and purchased a set of stainless steel bowls like the ones I kept seeing used in commercial kitchens on TV. Those things looked dented, bent, slightly burnt, as if they had seen action in the trenches of World War II. However, chefs still used them. Now I know why. They work, they are versatile and they last just about forever. I can mix stuff in them, stick them in the fridge, serve food in them, and even have my dogs drink out of them on a hot July day on the patio. They don't match anything in my kitchen. Think about this when purchasing a bench or a barbell.

Test It

Whenever possible, you want to try out the piece of equipment you are considering buying. Evaluate the quality, ease of use, and how your body reacts when using it (is the movement natural). This is especially important for cardio-based equipment such as bikes, elliptical machines, and treadmills, but is also an aspect to consider with bars, dumbbells, racks and accessory equipment. Don't be shy—you can visit sporting goods stores for this—then turn to cheaper outlets for the actual purchase if the store won't match the price.

Where is the Best Place to Find This Stuff?

So far, I've mentioned several places you can find good deals on home gym equipment, including sporting goods stores, mass market retailers, used sporting goods stores, and various Internet sources. In this section, I want to delve into more detail regarding coupling the strategy outlined above with the best time and places to obtain this type of equipment.

First, a few general guidelines.

- When obtaining home gym equipment, you have to balance shopping around with striking fast, especially when using online sites such as EBay and Craigslist.

- Don't be afraid of used equipment. There are entire continents of people who buy workout equipment, then stop using it and want to free up space—or just get rid of the damn stuff. Some of that stuff can be darn good to excellent. Often, gyms will put their equipment up for sale if they are upgrading or going out of business. When buying used equipment, be cautious—find out why the seller is selling. It may need repairs. Whenever possible, try out used equipment to ensure it functions and fits your body correctly.

With that out of the way, here are your best sources:

Friends & Family

Your friends and extended family members often have workout equipment—especially cardio equipment—gathering dust at home. Make them an offer. They may be glad to get some cash to get that thing out of their house.

Craigslist

For many, Craigslist represents the penultimate collection of used home gym equipment, especially if you live in or near a big city. This site typically has loads of used fitness equipment, because most people buy this stuff and just never use it. Thus, a lot of the stuff is 'like-new'. It can also be a trash heap. The real job is to sift through the junk and get to the jewels—like collections of bars, plates, benches and (yes!) racks. Often, you can find thousands of dollars of weights for pennies on the dollar. If the stuff you want is bundled with other stuff you don't want or need—and the price is right—just buy it. You can always use the three-pronged approach of garage sale, charity and landfill to expunge the extras later.

Additionally, the popularity of CrossFit in recent years has produced an interesting offset effect—obtaining high-quality barbells, plates and other free weight based equipment is now much more economical, because the supply has greatly increased, especially in this used, second-hand market (and as those novice CrossFitters come to the realization that CrossFit is a workout and not a training system).

Because of this, sites such as Craigslist (and to a lesser extent, EBay) have become dumping grounds for barbells, bumper plates and sometimes, Concept 2 rowers (do not hesitate!). Help the poor Crossfitters and take a barbell or two off their hands.

Your best bet here is to set up automated alerts (more on this below) as equipment you are looking for becomes available—because if you blink, it's gone. Then, evaluate and pounce. I've had friends who have scored entire collections of free weight training equipment (rack, barbell, plates, bench) in one shot for under $200. Those deals are rare, but set yourself up for success via automation and know what things should cost.

Used Sporting Goods Stores

I was able to outfit a good portion of my home gym by selling all of my old standard size bars and weights to Play It Again Sports and buy heavily discounted Olympic bars, plates and numerous cast-iron dumbbells.

Expect to find lots of Olympic bars, plates and dumbbell handles here, along with cast iron hex dumbbells. Typical prices will be in the 50-60 cents per pound range for the plates and bells. Remember, new prices will be around one dollar per pound and 45lbs is 45lbs. Things can be cleaned and painted.

You are also likely to find many orphaned pieces of cardio equipment. Much of this is of low quality and should be avoided. However, keep an eye out for AirDyne bikes, ellipticals or rowers. These air-powered machines are effective cardio units that hold up well over time.

I like to stop by my local Play It Again Sports about once a month—or at least quarterly—to see what 'new' stuff people have dropped off. I think that's a good general strategy for everyone, if you have one of these used sporting goods stores near you.

Amazon & Walmart

These guys are so massive that they can offer free shipping on most fitness equipment, including cast iron plates, power racks, and benches. I was able to purchase over 800lbs of rubber-coated cast-iron plates from Walmart.com with absolutely no shipping costs.

Amazon has many good deals on weightlifting equipment, but you have to look for them and sometimes wait (use the Wish List feature to monitor these items from a single place). Most of these deals are seasonal. Fitness equipment starts to drop in price, or have free shipping, right after Thanksgiving, when people are gearing up for their holiday purchases and planning their New Year's resolutions. Post-Christmas fitness sales are common, so make sure to browse the online stores after you've unwrapped your presents.

Finally, don't forget what Amazon was founded on—books. It's a great place to pick up books and videos for your training library, especially older, used books from Amazon resellers. Over the years, I've managed to add dozens of weight training and nutrition books to my collection at an average of $5 per book.

EBay

EBay offers a mixed bag of fitness goodies. But unless the seller offers direct pick-up and you live near them, you'll need to limit your searches to smaller items of less weight—unless your winning bid is so good that the shipping costs don't morph that 'deal' into a losing situation.

Newspaper Classifieds

Finding quality weight training equipment in your local newspaper or classifieds is sort of like waiting for Haley' Comet. All we know is that it's supposed to show up, usually several months after the New Year, amid the dead resolutions, but we don't know what may appear. If you normally get a daily newspaper, then go ahead and take about 30 seconds each day to look—otherwise, the sources listed above provide better returns for your time.

Garage Sales

This is actually worse than the newspaper. I'll tell you why.

First, you have to either look in your paper, read to see if any of the local garage sales list 'exercise equipment' or 'fitness equipment', or 'weights', or 'barbell', etc. Then, assuming you find something listed that is reasonably close, you drive there—and discover that it's already gone or it was the same sand-filled plastic weights you had at ten, including the cheap Weider adjustable bench that maxed out at about 200lbs capacity.

Alternatively, I shudder to think that you spend your Saturday mornings just driving around to yard sales looking for equipment. I can think of three things that would be a better use of your time, and they start with training, training, and more training.

If you do happen to find something of value here, you should be able to get it for next to nothing. The homeowners are looking to you as a trash haul service. If you need it, oblige them.

Other Sources

Besides Craigslist, Amazon, Walmart.com, and EBay, there are many dedicated equipment sites offering quality new and used items. For the budget-minded, start with UsedGymEquipment.com and go from there.

Forget about pawn and consignment shops. These places typically offer used equipment at prices that Amazon and Craigslist can beat any day.

Do-It-Yourself

Finally, if you have the time, patience and skills, many pieces of home gym equipment can be made from wood. If you have welding skills, you can turn out stuff that surpasses many commercial items.

Obvious candidates for DIY equipment include plyometric boxes and calf blocks. But you can also make effective and safe benches and power racks with a little more time and effort. The Internet is full of such plans.

• • • •

To sum up this section, the best places to find quality, effective and safe home gym equipment based on the variety of choices, price and the chance of scoring deals are, in ranked order: Friends/Family, Craigslist, used sporting goods stores, Amazon/Walmart.com, EBay, newspaper, garage sales. Consider DIY along the way as well.

A Trip to the Mecca—Not That Mecca

A few summers ago, my friend Jason was looking to buy some weight training gear to equip an employee workout center at his mortgage company. We discussed what he should get—benches, bars, plates dumbbells and a few machines—things I discuss in this book. He had a 2,000 square foot space (nice!). Now, we needed to figure out where to get all this stuff within a reasonable budget.

Because we both lifted for decades and live in Maryland, our destination was predetermined.

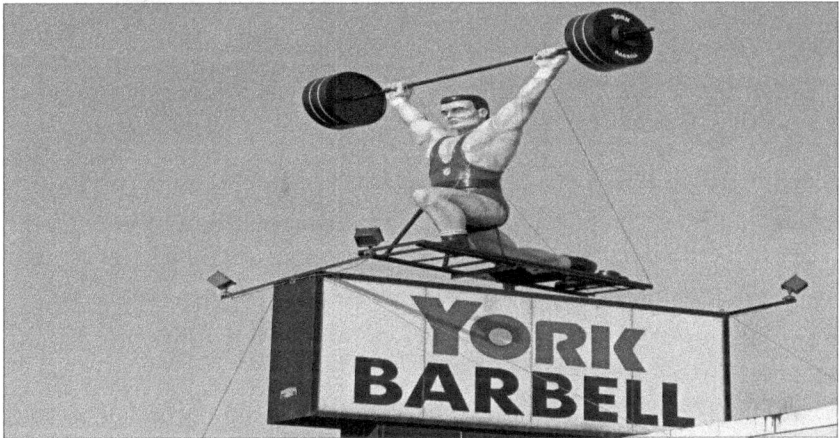

York, Pennsylvania is only a short 45-minute drive up Interstate 83. Lying at the end of those 43 miles was our Emerald City—the York Barbell Company. For most of us older folk, visions of barbells, cast-iron plates and quality mean one thing—York.

On a warm Saturday morning, Jason rented a large U-Haul truck and both of us clambered up into the cab, eager to visit the legendary manufacturing plant, warehouse and—bonus!—the USA Weightlifting Hall of Fame Museum, right on the premises.

Walking into the York Barbell Store with our list, we seemed to startle the employee staffing the counter, who was talking to his girlfriend on the phone. From his build, he was obviously a middle-aged powerlifter, with some clearly visible signs of muscle density.

"Can I help you guys?"

"Yeah, we want to get some equipment."

"No problem. Just look around and bring whatever you want up to the counter."

"Well, we have this list…"

He reached for the list, while still attempting to continue his phone conversation.

"Holy shit, I'll have to call you back."

Suddenly, the prospect of selling over $10,000 of equipment to two guys walking in off the street on a Saturday morning propelled us to VIP status.

"Guys, I'll need to call over to the warehouse—this is going to take a while. Hey, have you seen the museum? Let me show you something."

At that point, he lead us past the auditorium used for the World Weightlifting and Powerlifting Championships—the place where people like Vasily Alexseyev and Larry Pacifico competed on ABC's televised *Wide World of Sports* and NBC's *Sports World*—and into the famed York Barbell training room.

Now, this wasn't the legendary weight room, where Bob Hoffman of the AAU helped guide luminaries like John Grimek, John Davis and Steve Stanko—that was another time and place. No, this weight room was fully equipped for present day training. Power racks and platforms lined an entire wall. Barbells, dumbbells, benches, and cable apparatus seemed to be everywhere in this 10,000 square foot piece of heaven. Floor to ceiling windows lined the entire wall opposite the racks, allowing the bright Saturday sunshine to flow over the gloriousness.

Later, we were invited into the warehouse where they shipped all the famous York equipment to the world. Imagine the warehouse where they eventually stored the Ark of the Covenant at the end of *Raiders of the Lost Ark*—and imagine all those crates containing plates, bars, and dumbbells— as far as the eye could see. For some, heaven may be in Iowa, but for us that day, it was in York, Pennsylvania.

The point here is this—even if you aren't fortunate enough to live near a York Barbell, a Rogue Fitness or New York Barbells, you should still investigate to determine if there are any large weightlifting equipment supply warehouses near your location. You'll save on shipping costs (which can be high for things built out of steel and cast-iron) and be able to purchase new (or sometimes even traded in) equipment for manufacturers cost—eliminating markups to outlet centers.

How to Automate Your Equipment Search

Craigslist, eBay, Amazon and other web sites offer great bargains in both new and used equipment purchases. However, there are two problems here—time and timing. Sometimes it requires a lot of your time to look through all these sites to see if they have any good deals for a particular piece of equipment you want to acquire. I don't know about you, but I don't have a lot of free time to sit around and surf the net for gym equipment deals. Unless you get lucky and happen to search just as a good deal arrives (great timing!), you'll often find out about the deal after the fact. That's poor timing. I remember last year, when a pair of slightly used Cybex leg extension and leg curl machines went up on Craigslist for $300 each as part of a liquidation sale. Those commercial machines generally sell for $2000 each. By the time I saw the ad—hey, it was posted only a day earlier—those things were long gone. Great Craigslist deals wait for no one. Because most of us have lives, poor timing is often a common occurrence.

What we need is an automatic method that alerts us to those deals as they arrive. Most of us walk around all day with a smartphone, so let's use that to do all the searching and alerting. (If you only have a laptop or PC, this procedure will work for you as well—albeit with less convenience—so follow along.) What may take you fifteen minutes to set up can eventually save you hundreds of dollars. I think I have your attention.

There are many online sites and apps designed for info discovery and notification, such as Google Alerts, Yahoo! Pipes, and IFTTT. Perform an Internet search for things like 'Amazon price tracker', 'automatic Craigslist alert', etc., to find these useful servants. Use one of these to tell them what we are searching for and how to notify us. Once this is set up, the site or app will automatically notify you when the equipment you are looking for, at the price point you can afford, is available.

The Baseline Setup

In the summer of 1968, Frank Zane trained for his Mr. America and Mr. Universe victories at his St. Petersburg, Florida home gym. In two hundred square feet of space, Frank packed dumbbells, barbell, squat rack, dip bars, lat machine, preacher bench, and what he termed "a crude leg extension/curl". He also packed on a lot of muscle that year with that equipment, using consistently hard efforts.

Today, our baseline setup remains largely unchanged from Frank's collection. The purpose remains steadfast—we need equipment that allows us to lift heavier and heavier loads over time in relative safety.

Everything here centers on dumbbells, barbells and free weights—the time-tested tools of the physique gods. As you will see, choosing the correct set of dumbbells and free weights can be just as important as the workout itself—indeed, that choice determines the boundary of effort possible.

Therefore, our baseline setup includes the following equipment:

- Dumbbells (adjustable or fixed)
- Adjustable Bench (flat, incline)

- Olympic Barbell
- Olympic Plates
- Power Rack

The first thing you should notice is that this setup is similar to a typical powerlifters setup. That's intentional, because at the heart of every good bodybuilder is a powerlifter. The additional movements emanate outward from that, which necessitates the use of an adjustable bench instead of a flat bench, along with the use of dumbbells—the kings of movement patterns. You may also notice that the baseline setup does not include any pieces of traditional cardio equipment, such as bikes, treadmills, or steppers. This is also intentional, because we are talking about *baseline* setups. More on this later.

This baseline equipment allows us to perform everything we need to perform the basic human movements and build the complete physique:

Basic Human Movements	
Presses	shoulders, chest, triceps, forearms and abs
Pulls	back, shoulders, biceps, forearms and abs
Squats	legs, butts and abs
Hinges	back, legs, butts, forearms and abs
Carries	for just about everything, including abs, forearms, traps, spine, stability and systemic effect

A word on the carries—many bodybuilders neglect this type of movement. That's a mistake. There is a reason this movement has been a central component in all Worlds Strongest Man contests from the inception. In fact, they are so important to the development of core strength, and the muscles that resonate from that, that Stuart McGill calls these "moving planks". Remember, our goal is not to make narcissistic bodybuilders, but to develop the entire physique and to make men out of boys and real women out of ladies.

To get an idea of how many exercises can be performed with this bare minimum of equipment, take a gander at Bill Pearl's classic book, *Keys to the Inner Universe*, some time. As I thumb through that right now, it clearly illustrates over 500 exercises you can perform with those dumbbells, bench, and barbell.

Dumbbells—Minimal Investment, Maximum Returns

"I live temperately, drink no wine, and use daily the exercise of the dumb-bell."

--Benjamin Franklin, 1786

If you were a powerlifter, this is where I would say if you could only afford one piece of equipment right now, make it a barbell. Because you have bodybuilding aspirations, we need to alter this to say "dumbbell".

In fact, history provides our script. The dumbbell came first. Long before the barbell was first developed, the ancient Greeks of the 5th century B.C. were using "halteres", a crescent-shaped stone with a handle. These handheld weights were used as jumping aides and for exercises that included pushing, pulling, hinging and lunging. The first known haltere exercises were lunges, side bends and bicep curls. So, yes, the ancient Greek bros were curling from the onset. Perhaps Aphrodite was looking. And ladies, be aware that a 4th century mosaic from the Piazza Armerina in Sicily depicts Roman women using halteres for physical training—so dumbbells have always been an equal opportunity device. (The actual word "dumbbell" was coined during the Tudor period in England, where athletes used handheld church bells to train their arms and upper bodies. Because the bell's clapper was removed rendering them mute, they became known as "dumb" bells.)

Dumbbells are the simplest piece of equipment that allows us to effectively, safely and progressively overload our muscles through the five fundamental human movements (push, pull, hinge, squat, carry) in addition to opening the world of isolation exercises. Dumbbells allow you to perform millions of exercise variations, either bilaterally or unilaterally with a single arm—that's fairly hard to do with a barbell. Bill Pearl listed and described most of these in *The Keys to the Inner Universe*, more than three decades ago. So, if you get the dumbbells, get that book.

There are other benefits as well.

First, you don't need anything else—like a bench. We can use dumbbells standing or lying down, giving us tremendous variety of independent movement, hand positioning, and weight distribution.

Second, they are relatively cheap and take up little space. The amalgamation of cost, safety, variety and space make them the ideal first piece of equipment for the bodybuilding home gym. (There are a few disadvantages—namely, progression increments and positioning—but I'll minimize those shortly. Stick with me.)

Thinking about this more, dumbbells are a self-limiting apparatus. Looking deeper, Gray Cook, in his book *Movement*, describes the essence of this:

Self-limiting exercises make us think, and even make us feel more connected to exercise and movement. They demand greater engagement and produce greater physical awareness. Self-limiting exercises do not offer the easy confidence or quick mastery provided by a fitness machine...Self-limiting activities should become the cornerstone of your training programs...as movement authentication—to keep it real. The limitations these exercises impose keep us honest...

Dumbbells allow you to lift relatively safely. If you get stuck, you can drop them—this will happen and this will be a determining factor in dumbbell purchases, as you'll see.

The versatility of dumbbells is as astounding as the variety of body movements possible. Here's a quick snapshot of possibilities:

- Presses—floor press, kneeling presses, extensions
- Pulls—curls (supinated, pronated, hammer), rows, shrugs
- Squats—goblet squat, split squat, lunges
- Hinges—deadlifts, swings
- Carries—farmer, waiter carries

Now that you're convinced of the versatility of dumbbells, let's look at your options here.

Common Dumbbell Considerations

Dumbbells can be loaded with varying amounts of weight using three implementations—fixed weight dumbbells, adjustable, and selectable. This section will describe the advantages and disadvantages of each.

However, before delving into that detail, there are some common considerations that we need to apply universally to each of these types of dumbbells. These considerations can have a significant impact on how we can train with these implements.

Weight Range

Right now, your limit weight on dumbbell movements may be 40lbs. However, that's today and the name of the game is progressive resistance. Therefore, you need dumbbells that allow you to extend that limit as you grow stronger. Fixed weight dumbbells require you to purchase additional bells to extend this range. Adjustable and selectable dumbbells have a limit ceiling as to how much they can load or select.

Commercial gyms often have fixed dumbbells ranging in weight from 10-100+ pounds. Home gyms can attain this as well, although space availability may steer you towards a particularly type of dumbbell system.

Weight Increments

Traditionally, the big issue with dumbbell training, adaptation, and linear progression is that most dumbbells require five-pound jumps in weight increment. This may not seem like a big deal, but think in terms of percentage increases. If you can curl a 20lb dumbbell for ten reps and you want to continue adapting, curling a 25lb dumbbell represents a 25% increase in the load. That's a big jump.

This is an important consideration, not only at the novice level, but also especially for the seasoned intermediate to advanced bodybuilder. Making small weight increases is one of the keys to progress, regardless of exercise or apparatus.

For dumbbells, we really need the ability to increment the weight in 2.5lb jumps. For fixed dumbbells, this means either buying a lot more bells or adding micro-loading weights. Adjustable dumbbells can also use the micro-loading weights and prospective selectable dumbbell owners verify if those bells can increment in 2.5 or 5lb loads.

Commercial gyms may have dumbbells in 2.5lb increments at weights below 30lbs, but it's 5lb increments after that. Your home gym can dominate the commercial gym's setup here, and provide a superior environment for progress.

Collars, Clamps & Stability

Obviously, fixed weight dumbbells are fixed and secure (they had better be!). The same can be said of the numerous selectable systems. It's the adjustable dumbbells where we have to be concerned about how the weights are secured onto the handle, both for stability and safety. Again, there are several options here, including spin-lock handles (threaded to accept large nuts as collars) and clamps. Both can be effective if used and maintained properly.

The manner in which plates are secured to the dumbbell handle also affects how efficiently you can use them. Let's look at that.

Speed of Weight Changes

This is important for some advanced bodybuilding intensity techniques, such as drop-sets. Drop sets have been around since the invention of the dumbbell. However, those Greeks probably had a bunch of dumbbells lying around of various weights that they could quickly grab. Make sure, if you tread the path of the adjustable dumbbell that you can change the weight in less than five seconds or you can forget about the effectiveness of drop-sets as an intensity technique—and that's one less technique available to you in your hypertrophy tool belt. This becomes more important as you progress.

Although spin-lock dumbbells are safe and secure, all that spinning to change weights takes time. Sure, it's better than the old-school method of having a wrench lying around to loosen and tighten the nut on the dumbbell collar, but not by much.

The clear winner here is the set of fixed weight dumbbells, with runner-up status going to the selectable bells, which allow weight changes within that critical five-second period.

Maneuverability

Sometimes, the hardest part of dumbbell training is getting the things into position.

At relatively lower weights, it's not so much a problem. But, as you progress, get stronger and require the use of heavier and heavier dumbbells to continue progressing, a problem surfaces with adjustable, plate-loaded bells. I'm talking about the type where you load plates onto either Olympic or standard size handles and then attach a clamp.

In order to get heavier dumbbells into position—especially for any pressing movements—it requires a typical two-step process of getting the dumbbells to the ends of your thighs, then using those thighs to "kick" the bells into position. With handle-based, adjustable bells (especially standard size), this will be a painful maneuver, because the handle will be digging straight into your thigh. Fixed weight and selectable dumbbells do not have this issue, because they offer relatively flat surfaces at each end.

An additional consideration here is the length of the dumbbell as the weight increases.

An Olympic or standard size dumbbell handle is fixed in length. That means a 20lb dumbbell will be as long as a 40 or 60lb dumbbell. Long handles like this can force unusual movement patterns—think dumbbell curls where you want the dumbbell to start at your side with palm facing you—which may not be what you want and could cause compensatory problems as your body tries to adapt.

A typical fixed weight iron dumbbell of twenty pounds is approximately 9" long; its cast iron hexagonal cousin is about 11", whereas Olympic dumbbell handles are typically 20" long. Clearly, you can note the difference and the issue. Trying to supinate a 20" dumbbell handle with even a 20lb load presents problems.

Droppable (Can I Drop These Things?)

Regardless of your best intentions, you will drop dumbbells, whether through muscular failure, a slipped grip or perhaps to save your life.

Assuming we don't have to be concerned with the impact of the thing when it hits the floor (your floors are protected, right?), our next concern is whether the dumbbells can sustain repeated drops. This answer lies with the construction of the dumbbell itself.

Using iron plates on a steel dumbbell handle allows you to drop them repeatedly over time and by no worse for wear. However, as you move to fixed weight dumbbells, particularly hex dumbbells, as well as some of the selectable dumbbells containing plastic parts, thinking about dropping these things presents a dilemma—will it break (this time?) or should I try to resist and perhaps injure myself?

Space Requirements

Adjustable and selectable dumbbells were devised out of convenience and space considerations. It just doesn't take much space to store these types of dumbbells. Some models of selectable dumbbells offer weights from 10lbs to 120lbs in just two square feet of space. That's extremely space efficient, but comes with a much higher budgetary cost.

At the other end of the spectrum, having an entire set (defined by your needs) of fixed weight dumbbells requires lot of space. Multi-tiered dumbbell racks can help, but they will still take up significant amounts of space versus the adjustable and selectable varieties. I have a two-tier dumbbell rack with fixed weight dumbbells ranging from 10lb to 50lbs and that takes up nine square feet. Perhaps you can afford that cost.

• • • •

Each of these dumbbell considerations form an interplay of advantages and disadvantages that ultimately will determine the best system for your specific home gym setup and budget. There is no one clear choice that exceeds all others in all of the considerations. Sure, fixed weight dumbbells come closest, but can also require a hefty bank account to purchase and a small cavern to contain all of them. The point here is to make you aware of these considerations so you can match your goals, setup and budget to the appropriate choice for you.

Now, let's get into the details regarding each type of dumbbell system.

Fixed Weight Dumbbells

Fixed weight dumbbells are the most common type of dumbbell found in commercial gyms, where space is not a constraining dimension and speed of use is.

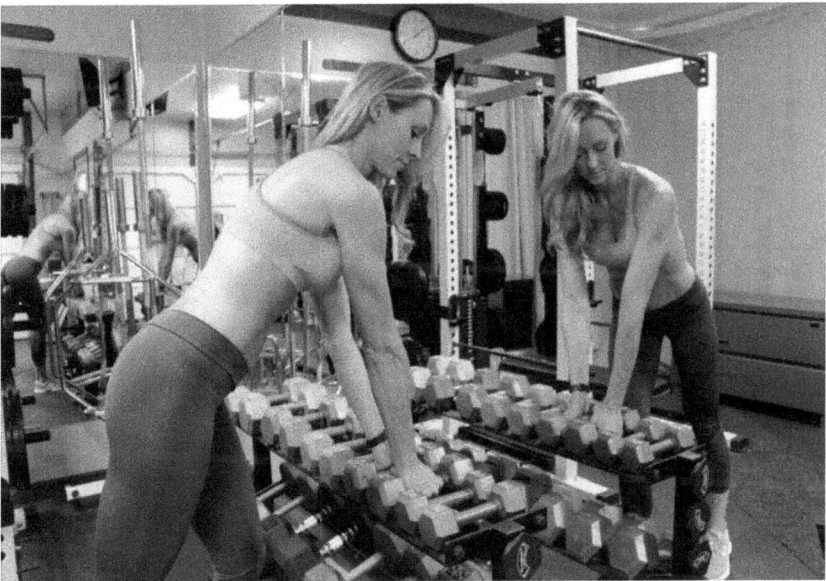

Acquiring a complete set of fixed weight dumbbells is the holy grail of bodybuilding. They promote rapid weight changes, can be dropped (if necessary) and are secure and maneuverable. However, there are two problems here—cost and space. A "complete" set is one that includes dumbbells weighing at least as much as you can handle for 4-6 reps. For many men past the novice and intermediate stages, that can be fairly heavy. I can handle dumbbells weighing in excess of 150lbs for 4-6 reps on shrugs, stiff-legged deadlifts, and one-arm rows. Many of the younger guys I train with routinely handle dumbbells up to 75-100lbs, especially after a year or two of consistent training under their belt.

So, assuming you acquire a set of dumbbells that match your proficiency level—at the typical five pound increment—that's a lot of dumbbells (assuming you start with ten pounders and go to fifty, that's already nine sets of dumbbells). At approximately $0.75-$2 per pound, that's both expensive in terms of cost and space. Multi-tiered dumbbell racks become a necessity with this system and they aren't cheap (unless you build them yourself).

However, you can acquire fixed weight dumbbells as you need them, which helps soften the budget blow and amortize the cost over a longer period.

If the fixed weight dumbbell system is the way you want to go, there are several types available. Let's explore the advantages and disadvantages of each type.

Iron Hex Dumbbells

This type of dumbbell is constructed using steel handles with the iron heads welded on. This is typically the cheapest option and the one most readily available, especially from used sporting goods stores. Note that handle thickness can vary here among manufacturers and models. Most hover around the 33mm width.

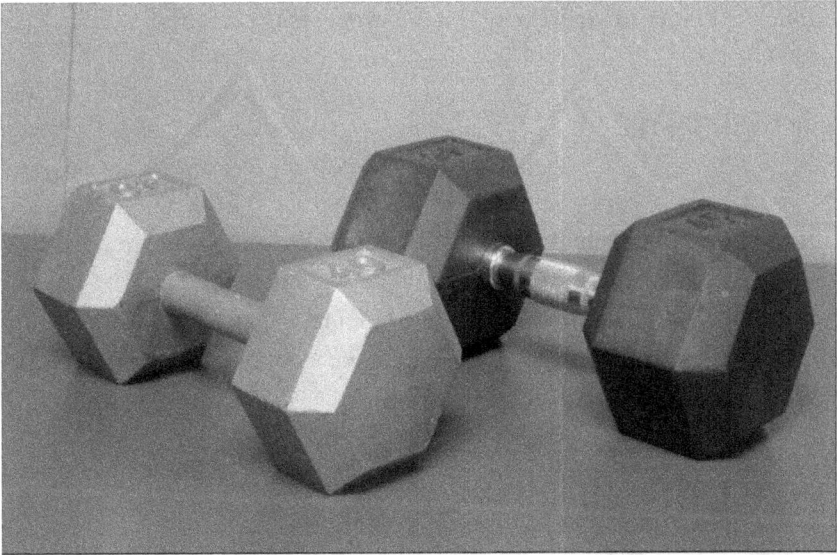

Once you get to the heavier weights here (60+ pounds) things start getting really expensive, they become harder to find and if poorly constructed, dropping them can end their life. I've seen 90lb iron hex dumbbells crack off the bell's head in some cases, even when dropped on thick, rubber flooring.

SIDE NOTE: If you have a pair of hex dumbbells, you also have your own push-up handles—as sold on TV. No need to buy the dedicated handles and one less item to clutter up your home gym.

Rubber Hex Dumbbells

One step up in cost from the iron hex variety. They also tend to be constructed with a higher quality than their iron-based brothers and include thicker (greater than 33mm) "ergonomic" handles, which forces your grip to the center of the bell. As bodybuilders, sometimes we don't necessarily want our grip there, especially with movements like supinating curls, side laterals and Scott presses.

Be aware that if you want to use PlateMates™ for micro-loading (more on this below), you won't be able to do it here, because last I checked, rubber doesn't contain a magnetic field. Of course, dropping a rubber hex dumbbell is kinder to your floor then the iron version. It's also a bit quieter.

Cast Dumbbells

This is the classic York dumbbell design, constructed from an integrated cast that includes the handle, making for a more durable bell. They are more expensive that the iron hex variety, due to this durability. I've never seen one of these break. If you're lucky, you may be able to find some of these on websites such as Craigslist, where the seller may not even realize the gold they are hawking.

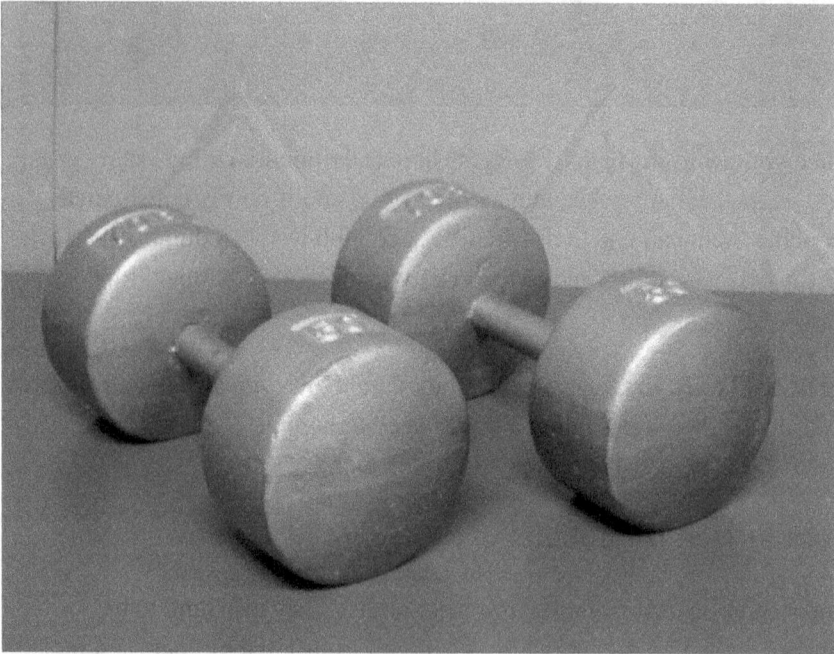

DIY Fixed Cast Iron Dumbbells

If you have the room, capability and time, making yourself a permanent set of fixed weight dumbbells using standard size plates is affordable. Noted strength coach Mark Rippetoe discusses the process of making dumbbells in this fashion—his Wichita Falls Barbell Club is outfitted with a set he had made over the years.

You'll need access to a welder and someone with welding skills for this project.

Here's the essence of this approach. Purchase a length of 1" diameter cold rolled steel for the handle assembly. I don't recommend the hollow steel tubes sold at most home improvement centers—because some of your dumbbells will be substantial in weight, we don't want to start with a compromised handle design. Next, get yourself some standard size plates in 10, 5, and 2.5lb sizes. You should be able to find these cheap at used sporting goods stores, yard sales, etc. Finally, get four large sized washers with 1" diameter center holes for each dumbbell you will make. Slide a washer on each end of the steel handle, followed by an appropriate amount of plates, finish with another washer at the end, and weld the washers in place. That's one dumbbell finished. Continue for as many dumbbells in as many weight configurations as you need.

PlateMates™ or Magnetic Attachments

One issue with dumbbell training is the load progression. After you get beyond the lower spectrum of dumbbell weights (5-30lbs), the load typically increases in 5lb increments. On the surface, this may not appear to be much of a problem, but it is. Think about the times you've hit a plateau with a dumbbell press. Maybe you were able to press the 50lb bells for 3 sets of 10 reps, but moving to the 55lb dumbbells represents a 10% increase in the load. Progression is often dependent on a series of small load increases, such as 1-5%. Obviously, we have a problem here.

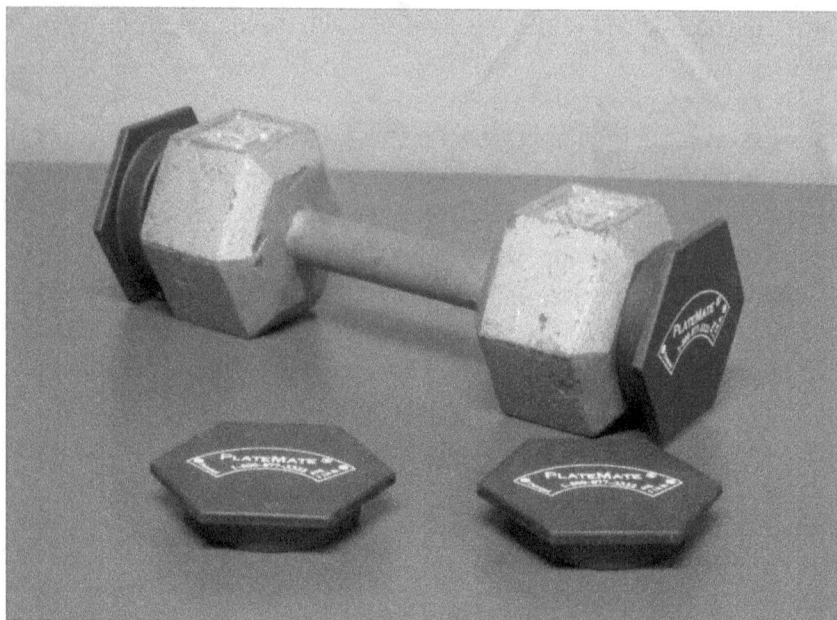

Magnetic attachments, such as PlateMates™ try to solve this, providing a 2.5lb load increase, instead of the customary 5lb dumbbell jump. Simply slap a 1.25lb PlateMate™ to each side of your dumbbell and you have instant access to every 2.5lb weight increment in your fixed dumbbell arsenal. And you just became a little more powerful.

There is one issue to be aware of here. Magnetic attachments add to the overall length of the dumbbell (about 1-2"). This can affect maneuverability and may cause you to alter your movement pattern on exercises where the bell travels close to your body, such as curls and presses. This is one of those instances where one to two more inches may indeed be too much. You'll have to decide.

Adjustable Plate-Loaded Dumbbells

The most economical dumbbell solution is the plate-loaded variety. Their biggest selling point is that a set of dumbbell handles and plates here can replace over 2,500 pounds of fixed weight dumbbells. That's a lot of dumbbells, space and money you can save. You already need plates (more on this later), and these same plates fit on Olympic-sized dumbbell handles with 50mm (1") sleeves. They come in several designs, which affect their usefulness.

Olympic Dumbbell Handles

Think of Olympic dumbbell handles as short barbells, with 2" diameter revolving sleeves. I don't recommend them for several reasons—the plates can slip off (depending on the type of collar you use—the stronger the collar the longer they take to remove for adjustment), the handles are 20" long (that means even 20lb curls will affect your form), and due to their length they affect many additional movement patterns, such as presses and extensions, etc.

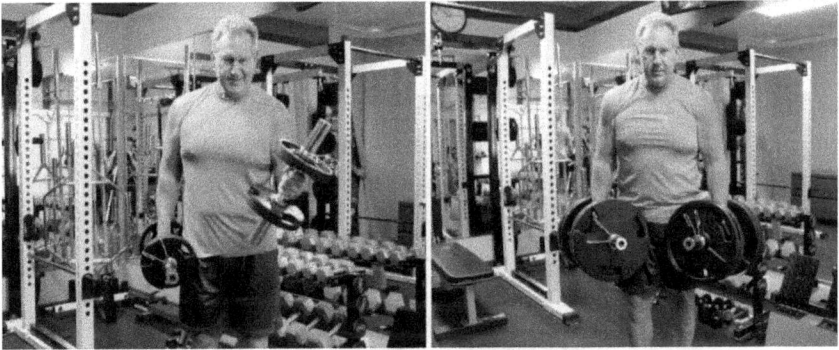

Other concerns include overall stability (safety) and the inability to use plates above 10lbs effectively, due to anatomical movement considerations of the wrist and forearm. Try curling an Olympic dumbbell loaded with a 25lb plate on each end. It's not pretty.

The type of collars you use can alleviate some of these issues. Lockjaw collars allow rapid weight changes, secure attachment, safety and confidence. Using spring-type collars is not recommended here.

Standard Dumbbell Handles

You may also want to consider using standard-size 3/4th inch diameter dumbbell handles (don't throw these away!), although these handles will limit the amount of plates you can use, due to their limited length (12"). A better option would be to purchase some ¾" steel pipe from your local hardware store, have them cut it to a longer length, and then slip a pair of standard dumbbell handle sleeves onto the pipe. This option, coupled with the copious availability of used standard-size 2.5, 5, and 10lb plates and some Lockjaw clamps provide a cheap, versatile set of dumbbells that you can load from 5 to 200lbs. The more pipe, handles, collars and plates you have, the more pre-set dumbbells you can have at the ready. The downside to this is you'll now have both standard and Olympic plates in the 2.5, 5, and 10lb range, so obviously dual-purpose use is out the window. However, you can extend this one step further, as Rippetoe has done at his Wichita Falls Barbell Club and have someone weld the plates onto the pipe/handle setup, making a cheap fixed dumbbell set, as I've described previously.

Threaded Handles (Spin-Lock)

Several online retailers also sell complete standard dumbbell handle sets with spin-lock handles. Because spin-lock handles are the same length as standard-size dumbbell handles, the same disadvantages apply.

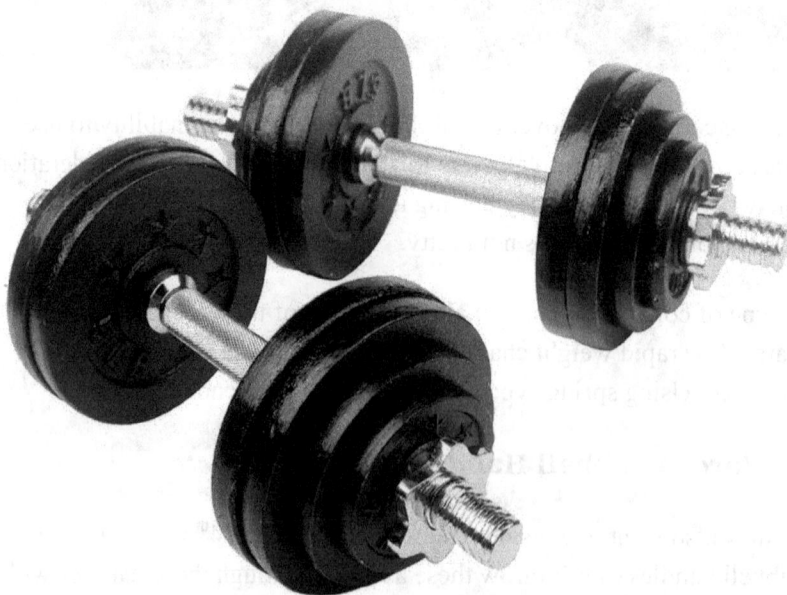

However, this type of handle greatly improves the speed you can change the weight and increases the safety, because the collar cannot simply slip off or work its way loose while in use. If you decide to go this route, make sure that you are purchasing a *set* of these dumbbells, because they are sold individually as well.

Pin-Based (Threaded)

Currently, IronMaster is the only player here. With this adjustable dumbbell design, special cast iron plates are loaded onto the handle and a threaded pin is inserted on each end to secure the plates. With various pin sizes, these dumbbells can be loaded from 20 to 160lbs, in 2.5lb increments, so capacity and weight increments are not a problem with this design.

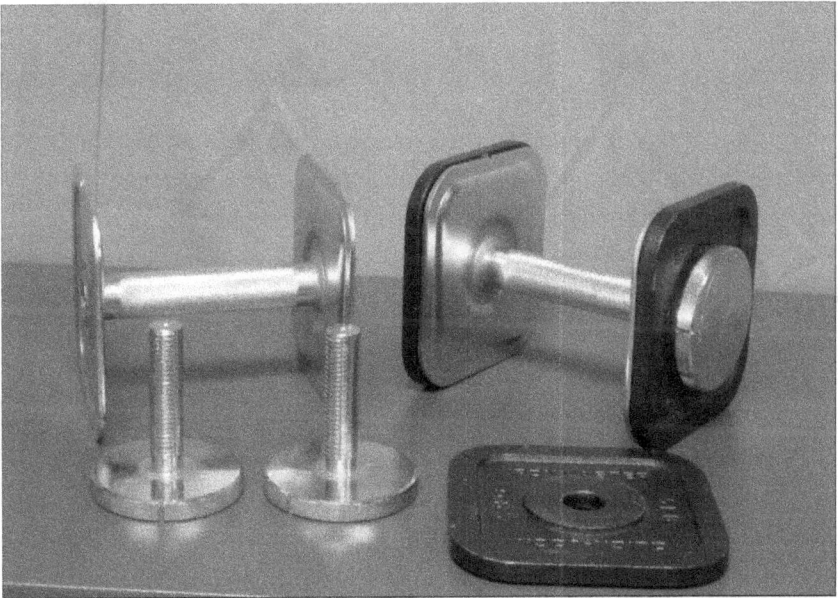

Weight changes generally take about 30 seconds per dumbbell—so forget about performing drop sets or any other rapid weight changes here. However, the resulting dumbbell is secure and feels like a fixed weight bell.

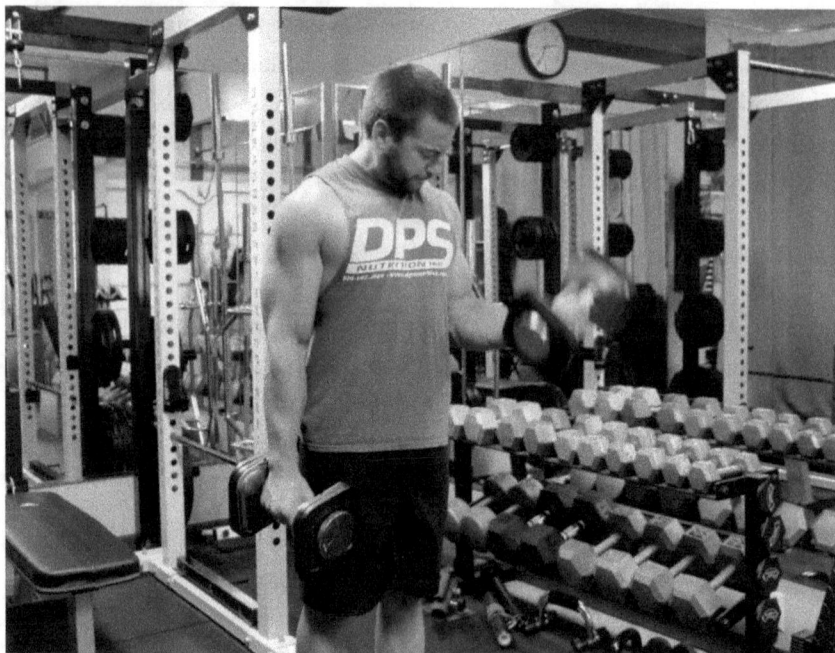

These things almost never appear on Craigslist (because they last forever and come with a lifetime warranty), so check the selling price and you may have found yourself one of the best deals in all of dumbbell land.

Selectable Dumbbells

Greg Olsen and Carl Towley created one-piece, adjustable dumbbells in 1991. Their design used a dial to adjust the weight and resistance level of each dumbbell. Today, Bowflex and Power Blocks are two examples of this type of selectable dumbbell. The benefits of this type of dumbbell system are size—they are compact (taking up about two square feet!) and typically include a stand—and rapid weight change. Both are convenience features.

However, be aware that some of the selectable designs include plastic and as such, come with much shorter warranties. Dropping them—especially repeatedly—may prove fatal to the bells. Additionally, some selectable designs contain that fixed length handle scheme, akin to the Olympic dumbbell handle problem, so pressing a 20lb dumbbell here has the same physical length as selecting 60lbs and pressing that. Think about that for your curls.

These are widely available on Craigslist—which may portend something.

Summary of Dumbbell Options

Here's a quick summary of our dumbbell options and how they stack up against each other.

	Fixed Dumbbells	Adjustable Plate-Loaded Dumbbells	Selectable Dumbbells
Weight Range	2 to 200lbs	10 to 200lbs	5 to 165lbs
Weight Increments	5lb (2.5lbs with PlateMates™ or if you are wealthy)	2.5-5lb	2.5lb
Maneuverability	Good	Poor (except for pin-based)	Moderate to Good (check the design)
Droppable?	Yes	Yes	Depends on design
Speed of Weight Changes	Instant	Slow	5-20 seconds, depending on design
Space Required	Can be substantial	Minimal	Minimal
Collars	None required	Spinlock or Clamp	Built-in
Cost	Can be expensive, depending on weight range needed	Relatively inexpensive (moderate for pin-based)	Moderate

Based on all this info, here are some recommendations. Unless you are buying a complete, selectable or pin-based system, you can acquire these as needed.

Budget Dumbbells ($50-$100)
Used, adjustable, plate-loaded dumbbells—standard-size or with Olympic handles.

Economy Dumbbells ($200-$400)
Selectorized or quick-change plate-loaded dumbbells. Get 'em used.

Luxury Dumbbells ($500+)
A complete set of fixed dumbbells. Get the wallet or the welding torch ready.

What did I choose? Because I already had a small collection of fixed hex dumbbells, ranging from 10-30lbs and a two-tier dumbbell rack that I obtained years earlier, I opted to extend this set of fixed dumbbells up through 50lbs, in five-pound increments. I was able to unload a bunch of standard-sized cast iron plates at my local used sporting goods store and used the store credit to buy the necessary cast iron hex bells. Now, fifty-pound bells may be good for women and many novice lifters, but they are mere warm-ups for me, outside of direct arm work. Therefore, I decided to bite it and purchase a set of IronMaster adjustable cast iron dumbbells from 20-120lbs. This combo, of fixed and adjustable dumbbells, allows me to perform quick weight changes at lower weights, yet still affords me the necessary stimulus for heavy, multi-joint work.

Now that you have the dumbbell options laid bare, those who opt for the fixed weight option need to consider storage alternatives.

Dumbbell Racks

Fixed dumbbells, especially a substantial collection of them, requires some type of storage rack in order to promote easy access and safety. The last thing you want to explain to your friends and family is how you were injured lifting—by tripping and falling over dumbbells strewn about the floor. I'm almost sure that's included in one of the thousand ways to die.

Enter the dumbbell rack.

We're not talking about those tiny vertical dumbbell racks that hold pink and blue and green rubberized "hand weights" between 2.5 and 10lbs. No, we want one of those one, two, or three-tiered horizontal racks, typically seen in commercial gyms that provide us with a space-efficient storage system for the home gym.

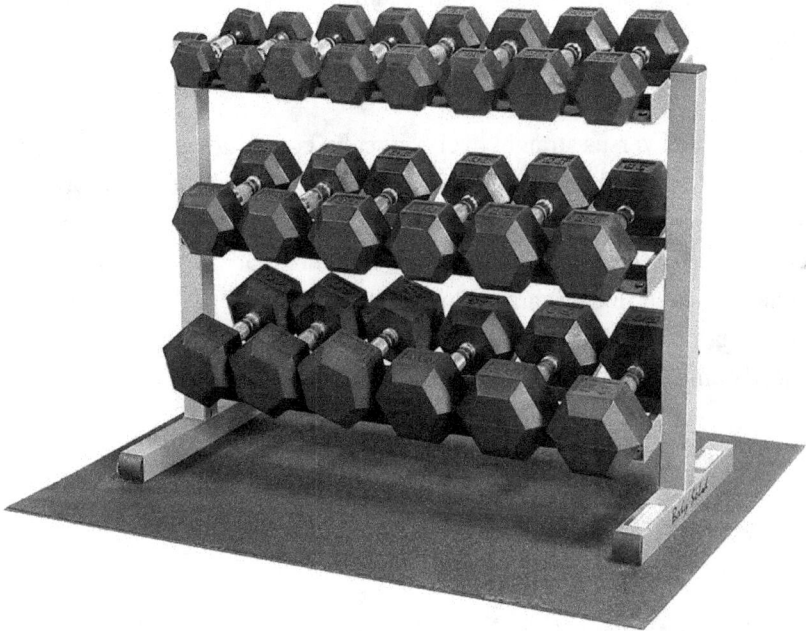

Multi-Tiered Racks

A lot of us start with our dumbbells stored on the floor. That works, until you trip and fall over the things or accumulate many dumbbells. Then the cursing begins. Dumbbell racks really help organize this situation and can save a tremendous amount of floor space, especially if you start talking about multi-tiered racks (two and three tiers). Typically, these racks occupy about 6-8 square feet of space—additional tiers occupy no additional space. Although most multi-tier racks are provided as a single unit, others are offered with a single or double tier, with additional tiers as add-ons.

Saddled vs. Straight

Most low-end dumbbell racks are built with straight rails—you can set the dumbbells anywhere on the rack. These go well with cast-iron or rubberized hex bells, because they don't roll. Higher end racks, like those in commercial gyms, contain cupped saddles for round, fixed weight dumbbells to sit in. Those are the gold standard, but again, you'll pay for that luxury and convenience.

So, the saddled versus straight decision really comes down to budget and the type of fixed dumbbells you own. Straight racks work for any type of dumbbell and are the least expensive. Saddled racks are designed for round, plate-based fixed dumbbells and are comparatively expensive. If you have uneven floors (garage floors have a slight slope for drainage), you may not want your round dumbbells rolling down the rack—if the rack is mostly empty.

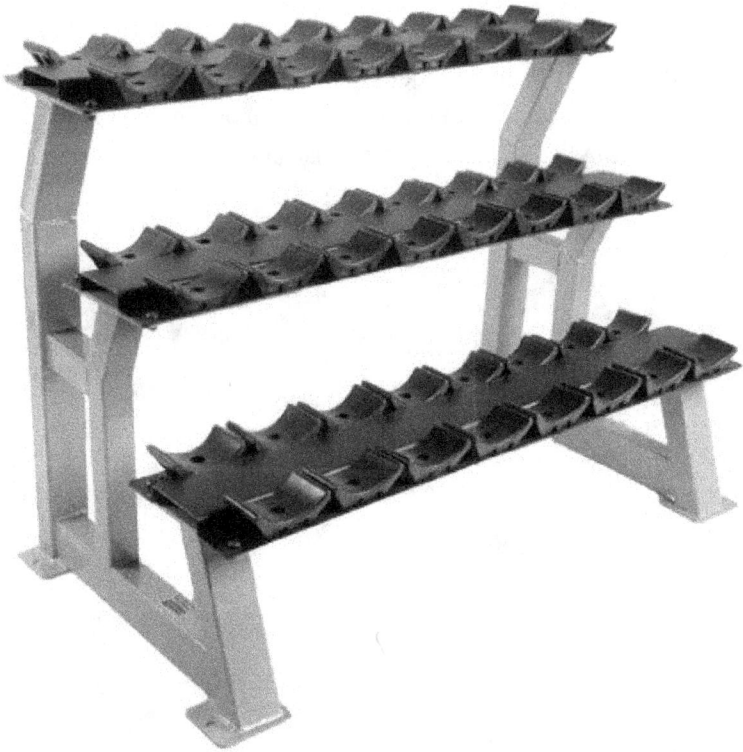

My two-tier dumbbell rack holds a set of fixed, cast-iron hexagonal dumbbells from 10 to 50lbs—all in a tight 18"x6' space. That's less than 5% of my garage gym's overall floor space, leaving plenty of room for activities. So, dumbbell racks make dumbbells not only effective and economical, but space-efficient as well. That's a trifecta for excellence in any home gym.

Dumbbell Exercise Movements

Now that you have your dumbbells—of any type discussed above—let's look at what you can do with them—without a bench. It should be apparent by the following list of exercises that this single piece of equipment quickly opens the universe of options.

Press	Pull	Squat	Hinge
Floor Press	Bent-Over Rows	Squats	Deadlift
Standing Press	One-Arm Rows	Goblet Squats	Romanian Deadlift
Flys	Upright Rows	Lunges	Stiff-Leg Deadlift
Extensions	Pullovers		Good Mornings
Standing Calf Raise	Curls		

And, because we are bodybuilders and tend to think in terms of muscle group specialization, here are the dumbbells exercises grouped by primary muscles affected:

Chest

- Floor Press
- Flys

Back

- Deadlift
- Bent-Over Rows
- One-Arm Rows
- Pullovers

- Good Mornings

Shoulders

- Standing Press
- One-Arm Press
- Lateral Raise
- Front Raise
- Bent-over Lateral Raise

Traps

- Shrugs
- Upright Rows

Biceps

- Curls
- Reverse Curls
- Hammer Curls
- Standing Concentration Curls
- Zottman Curls

Triceps

- Lying Extensions
- Standing Extensions
- Close-Grip Presses (dumbbells touching)
- Kickbacks

Forearms

- Behind Back Wrist Curls

Thighs

- Squats

- Goblet Squats

- Lunges

Hamstrings

- Stiff-Leg Deadlifts

- Romanian Deadlifts

Calves

- Standing Calf Raises

Abs

- Weighted Crunches

- Side Bends

And that's about all I have to say about dumbbells. Now, let's delve into the stuff that can take you farther than you ever imagined.

Plates—The Currency of Weight Training

Whether talking about dumbbells, barbells or even some types of machines, plates are the weightlifting currency that provides the progressive path to progress. In that vein, be sure of what you hold in your hand, for we seek not fool's gold and foolish purchases here, but the true plates of iron that will not fail you on your journey.

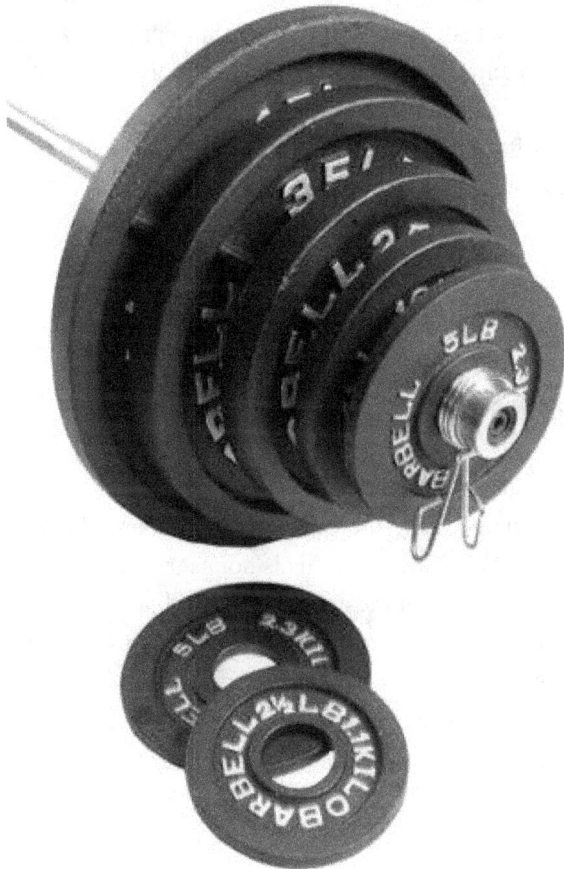

Here, we trade in cast iron with 50mm (2") holes. There are other considerations as well.

Common Plate Considerations

Don't buy the wrong plates and don't spend more than you need to. That's what this section is all about.

Size & Shape

For over a hundred years, barbell plates came in one shape—round. Then, someone who didn't know better decided to provide options here, and the hexagonal (or angular) plates were born. Their good intentions—hey, they won't roll on uneven surfaces—are anathema to proper barbell technique for movements requiring the barbell touch the floor, especially as the load increases. Angular plates make exercises where you pull the bar from the floor, like deadlifts and rows, dangerous. Not avoiding dangerous from the beginning is just stupid, so get round plates.

What about plates with handles cut into them?

Because that has no effect on performance, that's up to your preference.

Certified vs Non-Certified

Although musician and lifelong iron worshipper Henry Rollins has famously stated in his ode to the iron, that "two hundred pounds is always two hundred pounds", sometimes this is not as true as we would like. I've had college-age friends of mine actually notice that some of those 45lb plates felt "lighter or heavier" than others at their university gym—so they weighed them on a medical scale. Some were indeed 45lbs, others were 43lbs or 46lbs, and one unsightly character dared to be a measly 41lbs, even though he was obviously masquerading in the 45lb group.

What's the point of this discussion?

When you see a number stamped in the cast iron of a plate, your mind doesn't typically drift to question the validity of that statement. However, much of the world lies to you. Some are little, white lies—others, more damaging. Barbell plates are sold and advertised as either certified or non-certified for weight accuracy (if it does not state 'certified' then it isn't). Non-certified plates may carry the aura of white lies. Unless you have competed in sanctioned Olympic lifting or powerlifting meets, you've undoubtedly been using non-certified plates all along. Now, for those just getting the pump on at Gold's or trying to build some strength and muscle in their home gym, is this really something to be concerned with? Not really.

Certified plates will cost you double, or even triple, the cost of non-certified plates. As they say, we have bigger fish to fry here, so just get non-certified plates from a reputable company.

How Many Plates/How Much Weight Do I Need?

Based on experience, intermediate and advanced lifters have a good grasp of how much weight and how many plates they need—therefore; this is often a novice question.

Here's your answer.

In general, regardless of experience level, you need as much weight as you can lift and then a little more (this rule applies to plates and dumbbells equally) for progress to continue. If you are a novice, you don't yet know how much you can lift, so in this case start with about 300lbs in plates—that will take you from beginner through the intermediate stages of progress. For some, that may seem like a lot of weight—but remember, that 300lbs is spread across a menagerie of plate sizes.

Get the following plates (and quantities) at a minimum for a novice lifter:

- 2.5lb (2)
- 5lb (2)
- 10lb (2)
- 25lb (2)
- 45lb (2)

Of course, 'minimum' is relative to your current strength level. For proper linear loading, you need two of each type of plate (forget the 35s—you can substitute a 25 and a 10 pounder for that), so that's 175lbs of plates at *a bare minimum for a novice lifter*. Believe me, a male novice lifter with a couple months of proper training will be able to pull close to 175lbs off the floor in the deadlift. So, this is not as much weight as it may seem.

For the majority of intermediate and advanced bodybuilders, you will want to start accumulating plates toward this goal:

- 2.5lb (4)
- 5lb (8)
- 10lb (10)
- 25lb (4)
- 45lb (8)

This provides for proper loading and allows us to perform effective intensity techniques common to bodybuilding-type training, such as drop sets. It will also take you well into the intermediate to advanced stages of bodybuilding and strength training and gives up ready access to 400+ pounds for the big compound lifts, like deadlifts, presses and squats. Total weight here is 610lbs of plates.

Former Mr. Olympia Larry Scott also noted another issue with the amount of weight available, directly related to progress and ultimate achievement—he referred to it as the "fear of the biggest syndrome":

We can see this in every gym where the heaviest dumbbells are seldom used, regardless of what they weigh. Even the biggest guys will only use up to about 90% of what is available. That last 10% is almost always left to gather dust. This same "fear" limits us in our lifts, even if we are not even close to the heaviest weights available.

The morale and lesson of this story is always to have on hand more weights—whether dumbbells or plates—than you can currently lift. Experiment with Scott's parable. Equip your home gym with plates that exceed your greatest capacity by 20% or 30%. The crazy ones may opt for a 40% buffer. It's funny how the crazy ones seem to always move the bar upward in both society and the bench. You may surprise yourself here.

Once you have a firm grasp of the size, shape and quantity of plates you will need, you need to determine if cast iron or rubberized cast iron plates fit your needs and budget in order to estimate the cost of progress here.

Cast Iron

Cast iron anything is always cheaper than rubber coated because we are only dealing with one component and not two. Over time, that rubber will eventually wear away, whereas cast iron always remains.

Cast iron plates provide that "old-school" sound and feel. To us old-timers, there is nothing like that deep-throated rattle of three (or more) big plates on the end of a bar coming out of the rack. That can be a problem for those lifting in apartments, spare bedrooms or anywhere that noise reduction is paramount, wherever possible.

Some cast iron plates offer built-in hand grips ("grip plates"), promoting "easier handling". What is beneficial about grip plates is that those built in handles offer a tantalizing array of additional lifting options—using the plates themselves. For example, grip plates lend themselves to rows, laterals and carries, with no bar required. It's for this reason that I prefer this type of plate.

Typically, you can save money by buying a bar and plate package—
however, in most cases the bars are of low quality. Pre- and post-Christmas
sales (New Year's Resolutions!) are the best times to load up on these
barbell packages, because they offer heavy discounts versus buying a bar
and plates separately.

Rubberized Cast Iron

As discussed, this is a more expensive plate option than bare cast iron.
However, the noise reduction is significant, which is why most big-box
clubs and gyms have migrated over the years to this type of plate. If noise
reduction is a concern for you, then rubberized cast iron plates, coupled
with rubber flooring will go far toward meeting this goal. Consider the
rubberized grip plates here, as well.

Fractional Plates

Alan Calvert, the founder of the Milo Barbell Company in 1902, was quick
to note a common barbell and dumbbell issue evident even today in just
about every commercial gym on the planet:

*"The principle defect of bells that load only with plates is that they cannot
be increased in weight except in jumps of 5lbs or more. In order to
practice weightlifting safely and successfully you must have a bell that can
be increased one ounce at a time if necessary."*

Eventually, in your training you will reach a plateau where you can't seem
to increase the weight you can use on an exercise. One method to continue
progress here is through micro loading.

Micro loading is the use of small fractional plates in order to provide small
systematic increases in weight. For example, most gyms offer 45, 25, 10, 5
and 2.5lb plates. The 2.5lb plates are the smallest weight increment
available. What that portends then, is that you have no choice but to
increase the load on the barbell (or plate-loaded dumbbell) by five pounds.
That measly five pounds may be too much.

Because home gyms represent the pantheon of choice, with you as the owner/manager, get yourself some fractional plates and break free of this rigid loading scheme. Fractional plates can be obtained in 1.25lb, 1lb, 0.75lb, 0.5lb and even 0.25lb sizes. Although these fractional plates may lie around most of the time, they are a godsend for moving up in small increments when you are stuck at a weight.

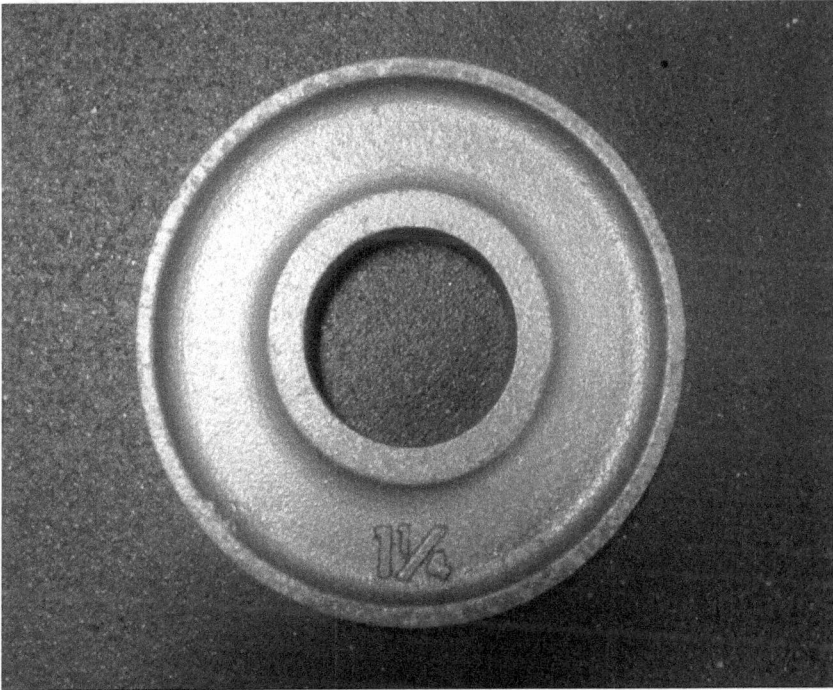

Just one problem here.

Remember our discussion regarding weights, plates and pricing per pound? Where a dollar per pound was a good baseline for obtaining new weights and half that for used ones? Well, because fractional plates also obey the laws of supply and demand, coupled with a specialty market, these things are expensive. It's not atypical to find a pair of new 1.25lb fractional plates selling for $20 or more. Now, my math skills are not the sharpest, but a quick mental calculation tells me that's almost *ten dollars per pound*. Yikes!

Luckily, equivalent results can be obtained on the cheap.

DIY Fractional Plates

Two-inch diameter washers and 20 oz. baseball bat weights are readily available, fit the barbell perfectly and are inexpensive. The 2" washers weigh exactly 0.625lbs each, so get yourself two for each side of the bar. They cost about $2 per washer, so you'll spend $10 to get fractional load increases. Not a bad deal. You can find these washers at McMaster or a Fastenal store, or just use the Internet to find a local source. Bat weights ("donuts") weigh 1.25lbs and are available in sporting goods stores.

Bumper Plates

What about bumper plates? You don't need them.

For those unfamiliar, bumper plates are high-impact, dense rubber Olympic barbell plates designed for Olympic lifting. These plates provide some bounce when dropped, thus sparing floors and tempering the noise. You see these today in CrossFit gyms.

Many a weightlifter and bodybuilder of old progressed quite nicely before the invention of bumper plates. Yes Virginia, you can lower a heavily loaded deadlift or clean without cracking the floor.

Because our bodybuilding training does not use Olympic lifting movements and we can lower heavily loaded bars to the floor, there is no need for bumper plates in a hypertrophy-based home gym. However, as Tommy Kono attests, there is great value in cycling between power and hypertrophy training. Mr. Kono was able to win gold medals in Olympic weightlifting in two successive Olympic Games, while also winning a Mr. Universe bodybuilding title smack between them. His famous training regime of 6-8 weeks of Olympic lifting, followed by a similar duration of bodybuilding efforts, kept both his body and mind fresh for new challenges.

Flip Kono's strategy on its head and maybe you do want a couple 45lb bumper plates lying around. If that sounds enticing to you, then you only need 45lb bumpers as your base, because you can add smaller cast iron weights that won't touch the ground for everything else. Optimally you should invest in an all-bumper set if you perform Olympic lifts regularly.

Plate Racks & Storage

In order to keep your home gym safe and organized, you're going to need some type of plate storage system, especially when dealing with limited floor real estate. Stacking plates on the floor, against the wall or in a corner may work for a while, but as you progress and your patience regresses, you'll see the need to build or obtain some sensible type of solution to the ever-growing plate problem. There are many options here.

Plate Trees

These things have small footprints, taking up about two square feet and can hold over 1000lbs of plates. Some models have wheels, allowing you to move them around the gym, but this is unnecessary. We're already in a smaller space and have legs and strong backs to move plates ourselves. If you don't, that's just another win-win. Less cost without the wheels and more physical work. Prices vary widely here, from a low of about $50 to upwards of $200 for the fancy wheeled versions. Used plate trees are quite common.

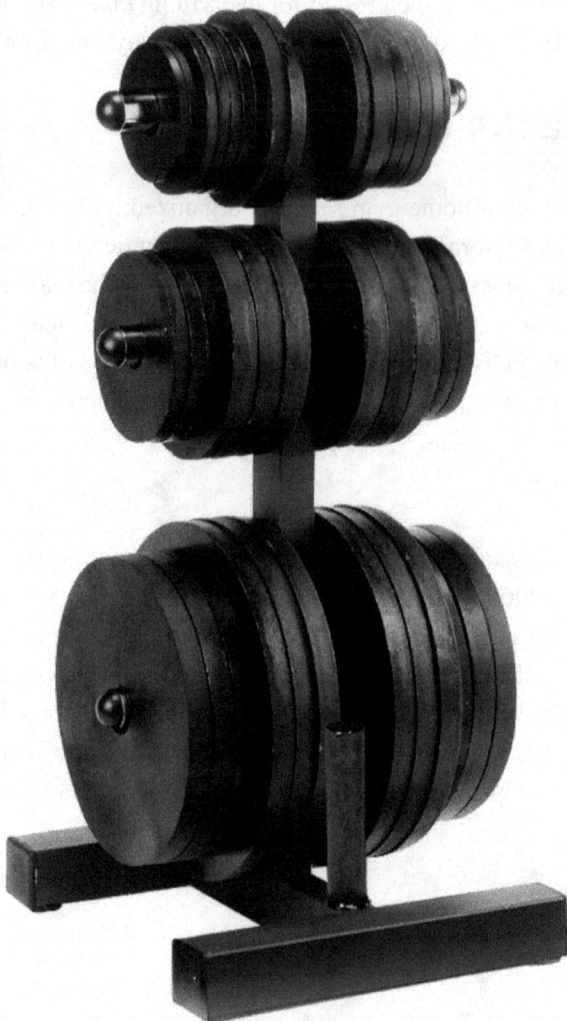

Horizontal Plate Rack

These are popular with Olympic and Powerlifters—in fact, you usually see one of them on each side of the lifting platform. The plates sit upright and are easy to get to (running a lifting event requires efficiency), the rack typically has wheels (some stationary models do not) and a handle for movement around the gym. Again, we don't need the wheels for our environment. If you go this route, make sure you get the appropriate type—there are versions specifically for cast iron and bumper plates. Expect to pay about $150-$200 for one of these new. Horizontal plate racks are not as common in the used market.

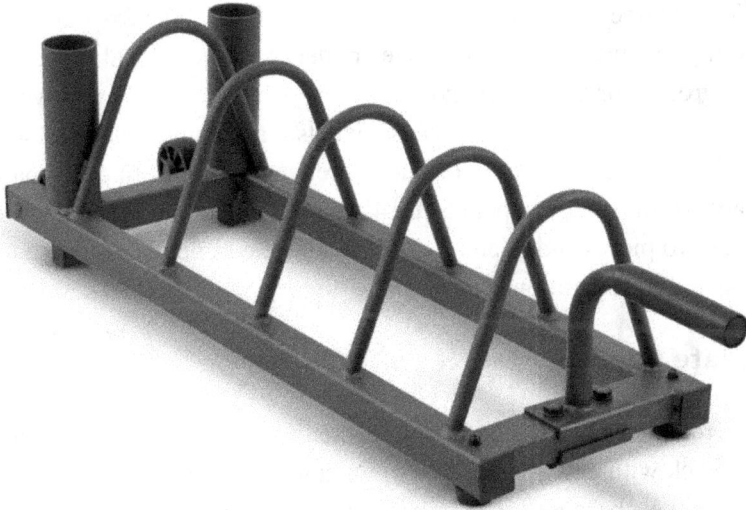

DIY Plate Storage

Because most commercial plate storage options aren't great feats of engineering, plate storage is one area that is ripe for DIY projects. There are several options here, each of which is cheap and practical to construct. Most of these storage projects should cost under $30 and take one to two hours of time. This could save you $50-$150 in commercial plate storage alternatives—money that you could use to buy plates.

DIY Plate Tree

This requires a couple 2x4s, some wood dowels and screws. Although the DIY version may not be quite as sturdy as its metal-based counterpart (don't try loading 1000lb of plates here), the benefit is that you may already have the scrap wood lying around.

DIY Plate Box

This is the poor man's version of the horizontal plate rack. A plate box stores your weights vertically in slots, making it easy to remove just the plates you want without having to remove other plates to get to them. Like the DIY plate tree above, you can assemble this from some 2x4s and screws. If you have access to a wooden pallet (go to your local farm, nursery, grocery or Wal-Mart and ask a manager if you can have a wooden pallet), things get even easier, because pallets make natural plate holders. If you don't have the floor space for the entire length and width of the pallet (standard North American pallets are 48"x40"), try cutting it in half and using the two pieces end to end—this provides the same plate storage in a longer space configuration.

DIY Plate Shelves

Multi-tiered plate shelves can be constructed with—surprise!—2x4s and screws. Stick with a two-tiered design for stability here. I'm not a big fan of plate shelves, because it just transfers the problem of stacked plates to a multi-tier setting. However, if you already have an unused or empty set of shelves in your basement, garage, spare room or shed gym, this may afford an opportunity.

DIY Plate Wall Hangers

Powerlifters have known the value of the board press for decades. Here, we are going to use the same concept of screwing together multiple boards—this time to hang your plates on the wall.

Use the studs on your wall to mount three 2x4s together with screws and 1" galvanized steel pipe (8" long for bigger plates and 6" for the smaller ones). Drill out the holes through the first two 2x4s, and halfway through the third (closest to the stud). Attach the first 2x4 to the wall stud using 3" lag screws. Attach the remaining two boards to the mounted 2x4 with 3" screws. Use a pipe wrench to screw in the pipe. Then, just hang your plates on the wall. This does get your plates off the floor, but does require wall studs and takes up some wall space.

Restoring Old Plates and Dumbbells

Several years ago, my next-door neighbor walked over to my fence and asked me if I wanted "these things". To the uninitiated, "these things" may have looked like some type of completely rusted WWII ordinance, but to me they were pure gold, especially once I noticed the word 'York' stamped into them. Two solid cast-iron York 50lb dumbbells—free of charge.

Old weight sets are a common item at many garage and yard sales. If you come across a set of plates or cast iron dumbbells that you need—but are covered in rust—there is a good chance you can bring them back to life with minimal effort and cost. Using the procedure I'm going to describe below, I was able to restore those old York dumbbells back to a "like new" state.

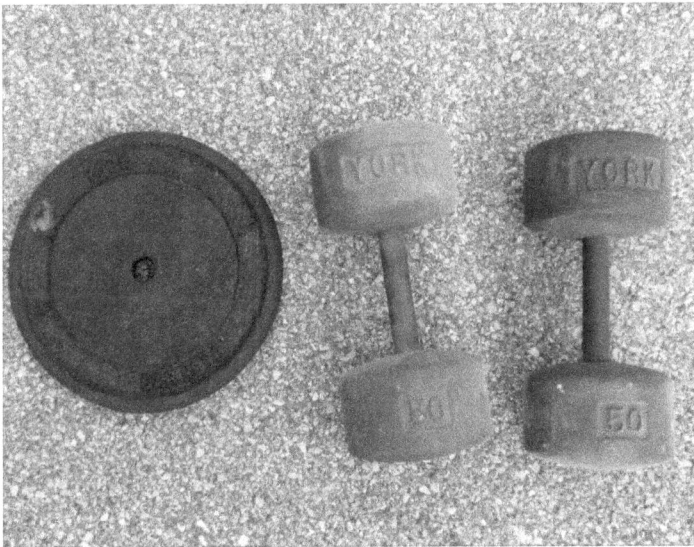

Here's the procedure.

Clean the weights with water, using a hose and wire brush to remove any loose rust and grime.

Dry the weights and place them in a large container filled with Coca-Cola. (Coke contains phosphoric acid, which is what removes rust.) Leave them there for at least 3-4 days. If minimal rust remains after this time has elapsed, you can skip directly to the final touches below. If you are short on time or patience, use naval jelly (phosphoric acid in much higher concentrations than Coke) which will reduce the time required from several days to about ten minutes. If you go that route, you'll also need to use some appropriate gloves and mask for safety.

Remove the weights, spray them with a hose and use the wire brush again to remove any remaining rust loosened by the soda. You can also use WD-40 to assist this process.

Finally, finish the weight restoration by spray-painting them with quality rust-stop paint, such as Rust-Oleum, Eastwood Rust Encapsulator or POR-15. You want to use a paint that chemically locks in any remaining rust so it won't spread. Check with your local auto parts store—they typically deal with the restoration of car parts, and can provide you with some good options here. I like to use either a gray or a black paint with this step, matching the color with my other weights.

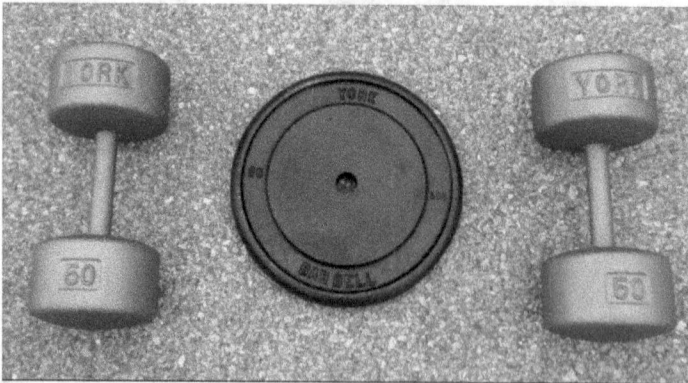

Summarizing our plate options, here are my recommendations, based on a 300lb set of plates.

Budget Plates ($50-150)
Buy used cast iron plates. Pay no more than .50/lb or this won't be a budget deal. Stack the plates for now, or build yourself a plate storage solution.

Economy Plates ($150-$350)

Buy cast iron or rubberized cast iron plates from a large retailer (think Walmart). Free shipping really helps here. Buy some large washers for your fractional plates. Get a plate holder from a used sporting goods store.

Luxury Plates ($350+)

Buy new, cast iron or rubberized grip plates and a complete set of micro loading plates. Get them all from the same manufacturer so they are uniform in appearance. Buy a high-capacity plate holder. Let your friends admire, then get to work.

Benches

A bench allows you to expand your floor-based or standing presses into a bench press and allows you to add pullovers, step-ups, and many other movement variations. An adjustable bench further expands this scope to include incline presses, fly, extensions, and more. Let Bill Pearl's *Keys to the Inner Universe* guide you here.

Legendary strength coach Bill Starr summed up the importance of bench selection in *Only the Strongest Shall Survive* when he wrote, "a strong solid bench is not a luxury, but rather a necessity if safety is honestly considered."

Size, Stability & Capacity

You'll need a bench that is sturdy, solid and heavy-duty, rated at holding at least 500 pounds minimum (1000 pounds is ideal—remember, you and your progress are a moving target—over time, you'll weigh more and move more weight). Don't forget, that capacity number also includes your own body weight, so gauge from there. Make sure the bench does not move or wobble when in use.

Beyond sturdiness and capacity, weight-training benches also need to be of proper length, height and width. Because I've yet to see a bench I thought was too short or long for my average male height of 5'9", only you can make that call. If you stand eye-to-eye with Shaq, then you already know what to look for here. More commonly, make sure the bench isn't too wide—I've seen some benches that are wide enough to interfere with the natural movement of arms and shoulders in the bottom position. Adjustable benches are notorious for widening the short bottom portion of the bench, especially if they accept attachments (more on this in a minute). If you make an impulse buy on a bench that's too wide without testing it, you'll regret it every time you use it.

For comparison purposes, the standard size (most common) for a weight-training bench is 19" high and around 42" in length. Benches taller than this may not provide the ability for you to keep your feet planted firmly on the floor—an aspect that becomes evident in importance as the load increases.

Another stability factor is the density of the foam under the bench's covering. Like any truthful college coed will tell you, harder is better. Look for high-density foam, where 2" thickness is ideal.

The final piece of the stability equation is the size of the bench's steel tubing (legs and frame support) and the feet. Pay particular attention to the feet—you don't want this thing moving when you are under load. Heavy, rubber feet are the gold standard. High-quality, high capacity benches are typically constructed with 2"x2" steel framing. Consider the bench you are contemplating and compare to that number.

Now that bench size, stability and capacity are considered, the functionality of the bench becomes important, determining how far you can extend the scope of exercise movements. You have two choices here—flat utility benches and all-in-one adjustable benches. Let's look at each.

Flat Utility Benches

Flat benches that don't adjust are the juggernauts of the pressing world. They are veritable bastions of stability (at least good ones are), built to withstand big bodies with big pressing loads. That is their greatest strength.

Although the bodybuilder can certainly use these for a myriad of movements, such as presses, pullovers, extensions, flys, and curls—to name a few—they offer but a single angular plane from which to originate. Sure, you can prop up one end or the other with a plate under the bench's feet, but that only gets you so far in the incline or decline world—and the world of angular stress vectors is what much of bodybuilding is about.

Therefore, if you do get a flat utility bench, get it after you have a good adjustable bench.

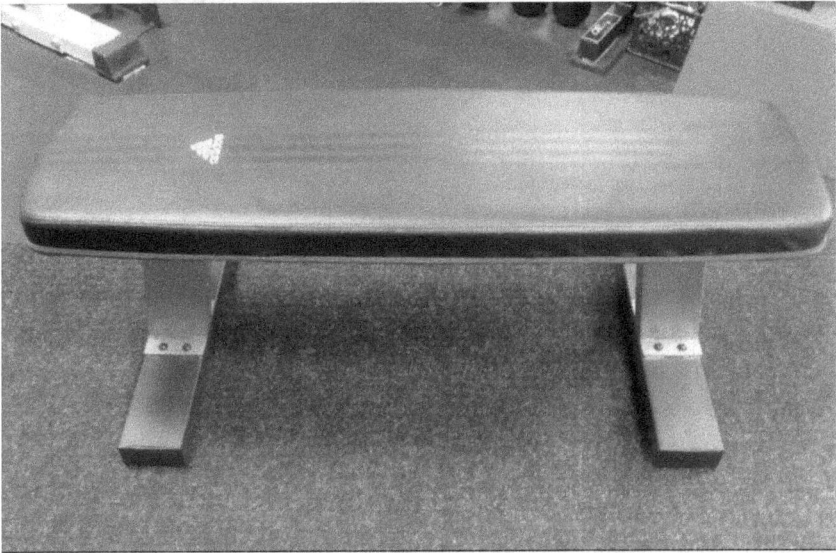

Adjustable Benches

This is what the bodybuilder is looking for in bench versatility—a single bench that does multiple duty through various incline—and perhaps—decline angles.

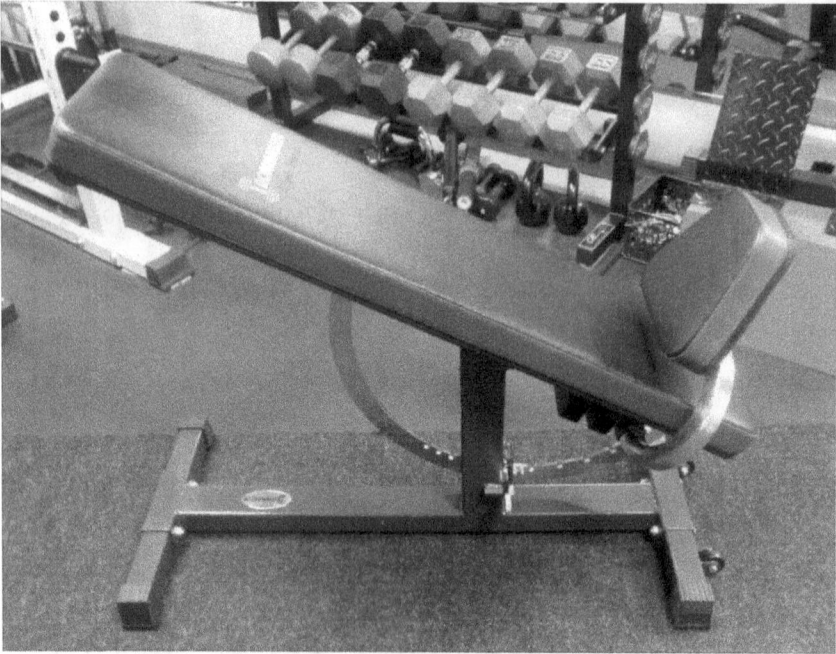

The important considerations here are the number of angles available, the seat, moving the bench around, and finally—attachment options. Let's look at each.

Adjustment Angles

In general, for a bodybuilder the number of adjustment angles the bench offers, the better. Notice the speed and ease of adjustment. Advanced overload techniques, such as angular drop-sets demand quick angle adjustments. This thing also needs to go from flat to vertical. Make sure it doesn't stop short of that vertical—otherwise you may find yourself needing an additional bench.

Additionally, check to see if the seat portion of the bench can be independently adjusted from the rest of the bench. This can be important, because an unyielding, horizontally-set seat, coupled with a low incline bench angle can find yourself sliding off the seat at worst, and in most cases reducing pressing power by creating an unstable base.

What about decline angles? I wouldn't worry. Decline pressing is overrated, ineffective and hubris-based, compared to your real alternative—weighted dips. We'll get to that shortly.

The Seat

A good friend of mine bought a nice adjustable bench with many adjustment options—including independent adjustment of the seat angle—and the ability to add lots of attachments. There was only one problem. The seat was wider—much wider—as it approached your knees. Now, I'm a fairly big guy, but this bench was like sitting in one of those leg adduction machines at the gym. Except I'm not doing leg adductions. I'm just trying to sit and concentrate on the lift, not be preoccupied that my groin area has been spread wide open.

Make sure the seat is comfortable and fits you well. You're going to be spending a lot of time sitting on this under load.

Moving the Bench Around

Typically, adjustable benches are heavier than most flat utility benches. Because you'll be moving this thing around a lot—is that energy expenditure part of your workout?—you may want to consider a unit that has integrated wheels at one end of the base for easy mobility. It's a small thing, but one that can make life a lot easier, especially if younger kids will be using this or just trying to get it out of the way for some floor-based exercise.

Attachment Options

Because home gyms offer limited space (and budgets), an adjustable bench that accepts various attachments, such as a leg extension/curl and preacher curl becomes a valuable commodity. A quick warning here—don't get a bench that has either of these two curl-based devices permanently attached. It must be removable or will get in the way of proper foot placement for presses and just about anything else other than leg extensions and curls. Remember when car phones were permanently installed in cars by the manufacturer? Yeah, we don't want to repeat that mistake.

Dumbbell Exercises with a Bench

By adding an adjustable bench, you expand the scope of exercises that you performed on the floor with dumbbells to include the following:

- Step-Up
- Seated Calf Raise
- Bench Press
- Incline Press
- Decline Press

- Incline Fly
- Decline Fly
- Bench Row
- Seated Press
- Bench Shrug

- Preacher Curl
- Incline Curl
- Incline Extensions
- Wrist Curls
- Wrist Extensions

There are many more. Let Pearl's book guide you here.

Prices on flat and adjustable benches may represent the widest spectrum of cost derivation than any other type of weightlifting equipment. You can find good, solid adjustable benches at garage sales for as little as $50 or new on the Internet for about $150. And you can also find them for close to $1000. The biggest characteristic in price variation is bench capacity and construction.

Budget Bench ($50-$100)
A used adjustable bench that accepts attachments (leg extension/curl, preacher curl). Just about any will do here as long as it's stable and matches your current capacity.

Economy Bench ($100-$300)
The only difference here from the budget models will be the bench capacity and durability. Bigger, stronger guys may want to start from here.

Luxury Bench ($300+)
Two benches—a flat utility bench and an adjustable bench. Both should be high capacity (600+ lbs) and built like tanks.

Barbells—The Key to Maximum Development

The barbell excels where the practicality of dumbbells end. The barbell is the nucleus of the home gym and the central implement for long-term change. You can train everything with a barbell using an almost infinite level of loading—or at least a level that your genetics, drive and desire ultimately dictate. You can also micro-load as little as a single pound or less and lift loads that no dumbbell can accommodate. That drives adaptation.

The original barbell was invented during the 19th century in Europe, whereas the modern cast-iron loaded variety came along during the early 20th century with the founding of the Milo Barbell Company in 1902. The modern barbell used today has not fundamentally changed since the 1928 Olympic Games when the Berg revolving barbell sleeve became standardized.

The world of barbells, and their corresponding plate brethren, are split into two pantheons—Olympic and Standard.

Standard (or "regular") barbells are one-inch diameter steel shafts with no rotating sleeves—they don't allow the weight plates to rotate freely, meaning the barbell will always be trying to rotate out of your grip, peeling your hands open. This type of bar is great for your forearms and for working out when you're about ten, but bad for everything else you're trying to do to get stronger and more muscular. Standard bars also begin to bend when loaded beyond 200lbs. You see these bars at Sears, Walmart, most garage sales and in the sand-filled days of your youth. Avoid these or your progress will eventually grind to a halt and your bar and plate acquisition odyssey will need to start anew.

'Olympic' barbells have sleeves that rotate freely on either side of the bar. The York Barbell Company originally manufactured these types of barbells, used for the first time at the Olympic Games in Amsterdam in 1928, starting in the 1930s. Regulation Olympic bars are seven feet long and built for heavy lifting. They are common in high school and college gyms and every commercial gym. You want an Olympic-size bar and the Olympic-sized plates to load on it for your home gym.

Once you get the differences between Olympic and Standard bars sorted out, the varietal world within Olympic barbells emerges. The remainder of this section will give you an understanding of what to look for when choosing an Olympic barbell and what kind of bar is best for bodybuilding-type training. Because the barbell is so central to your training, you don't want to choose the wrong bar, or—even worse, the right piece of crap.

The first thing you need to think about for your home gym is just who is going to use a barbell and for what purpose. Is it just you, or are your husband/wife and any kids going to work with it? There are differences in barbells for men, women and youth, varying in weight, shaft diameter and length.

Men's Olympic and Powerlifting Bars

Almost all barbells you've probably encountered are men's powerlifting bars. The difference between an Olympic lifting bar and a more traditional power bar are in the shaft diameter, knurling, and the flex/whip effect. The common specs here are a weight of 20kg (45lbs) and a length of 2.2 meters (a bit over 7ft).

Olympic lifting bars traditionally have shaft diameters of 28-29mm (28mm is the official International Weightlifting Federation specification), no center knurling, light shaft knurling and medium whip/flex for performing the Olympic lifting moves (the snatch and clean and jerk). Typically, they contain ring marks for both Olympic lifting and powerlifting.

Powerlifting bars, found in almost all gyms, are much more rigid beasts, used for slow, heavy lifts (think presses, squats and deadlifts) where we desire minimal bar flex. These barbells sport shaft diameters from 28-32mm, medium knurling in the center (for securing squats and front squats) and additional knurling all the way to the collars to offer secure gripping anywhere. For bodybuilders, as Obi Wan would say, "these are the bars we are looking for."

Women's Bars

Olympic lifting barbells designed specifically for women weigh 15kg (33lbs), have a shaft diameter of 25mm and share the same length as the men's bars. In essence, they are lighter and designed for smaller hands.

Training Bars

These are Olympic bars of varying lengths (60", 72"), diameter (25mm, 28mm) and weight (8lb, 15lb, 10kg) primarily used to train novice users or for perfecting technique.

Youth Bars

Olympic lifting barbells designed specifically for youths weigh 10kg (22lbs), have a shaft diameter of 25mm and a shorter bar length ranging from 60-67 inches (about 5-12 inches shorter than the men's and women's bars). The length reduction is due to shorter sleeves, thus less weight can be loaded. The astute connoisseur of weightlifting will note the systematic changes in bar weight of 5kg between the men's, women's and youth barbell varieties. Clever humans.

In case you don't understand what difference shaft diameter makes or even what knurling is or does, let's take a look at all the aspects of barbells so you can make informed, intelligent choices here.

Characteristics of Barbells

Certified vs. Non-Certified

A certified bar conforms to the Olympic barbell specifications from the International Weightlifting Federation (IWF). Certified bars also guarantee the weight of the bar is exactly as advertised (in international weightlifting competitions we can't have any variations between bars or political incidents may ensure—god forbid a non-conforming barbell would start the next world war. I'm joking, I hope.)

In any case, for bodybuilding, we don't need to concern ourselves with certified or non-certified bars. There are more practical considerations, which we'll get to next.

Tensile Strength, Steel & PSI (Load) Rating

All of these various terms concern the breaking point of a barbell. Yes, barbells can break, although the chances you'll ever do the breaking is slim. What is more likely is that you might permanently bend the bar by dropping it on the floor or the power rack's safety rods/rails with a heavy load—so don't do that.

Our concern is with how heavy the load can go before this happens. Here's all you need to know—look for the PSI or load rating. You want to see a number that is 150,000 or greater. If the rating is less than that—or worse—there is no rating, skip right on past that bar. Cheap, mass-market bars typically have PSI ratings of 65,000 (yikes!). Great bars are at 200,000 or above. More specifically, PSI ratings from 90-130,000 are low-end bars that are rated to hold 500 to 1,000lbs before breaking. That's not much, especially if you factor in the force applied to the bar in addition to the load. (Take a 500lb rated bar and try a 500lb clean & jerk on it—it will snap like a twig.) Mid-range bars have PSI ratings from 130,000 to 160,000 (1200 to 1500lbs), whereas high-end bars are above 160,000 PSI and can easily handle 1500+ lbs of load plus force. My advice—take the route of the middle bear in Goldilocks and gravitate toward the mid-range bars for bodybuilding—not too crappy, not too expensive—just right. These mid-range bars should last you a lifetime. Coincidentally, they are also the bars you'll find in just about every gym, health club and fitness center in the world. High-end bars live in black iron, serious powerlifting or Olympic lifting gyms.

The bottom line is this. Weigh the price and condition of the bar against the rating (or lack thereof). If you're in a second-hand sporting goods store and they are asking $50 for the bar that has no discernable defects (bolt sticking out of the sleeve, slight bend, etc.), and no way to know the PSI (don't even ask), then go for it.

What did I do when first outfitting my home gym? I bought a new $99 bar from an online retailer and quickly regretted it. Not just for the sausage-like feel of the 32mm diameter (I'm used to 28-30mm from 25 years in commercial gyms), but for the light knurling and weakness of the bar, especially when I'm pulling heavy deadlifts. Now, for novices or those with limited funds, this is ok, but not for advanced trainers who have climbed up the load ladder. I had to go out and get a reputable, mid-range bar.

Bearings & Bushings

Bushings and bearings are what allow the sleeves on the barbell to spin on the shaft. Bushings are low friction, whereas bearings provide even less friction, allowing the sleeves to spin much more smoothly, something that's important to explosively powered Olympic lifting. This comes at higher cost (bearings are more difficult to manufacture). Because we are concerned with hypertrophy-based training, the bushing-based bars are fine for our purposes. That's a good thing, because it keeps our cost down here.

Length

We've already discussed this, so to summarize the length is typically 7ft, but can also be 6ft and 5ft. I'll discuss the shorter varieties in the Specialty Bars section below. The seven-foot bar is your prime implement of mass construction.

Bar Diameter

Again, we've already touched on this, so here's a quick summary. The diameter of a bar affects the stiffness and how much "whip" it produces on a lift. Diameters of 28mm are common for Olympic weightlifting (it's the spec) and CrossFit, whereas 30-32mm is commonly used for powerlifting and bodybuilding. If you only buy one bar for varied purposes, a 30mm bar is probably best. Be aware that many cheaper bars (32mm raise your hand) are thicker in diameter due to inferior steel which cannot remain straight at 28mm. Adding some thickness makes them stronger.

Knurling Markings (Placement), Depth & Length

Knurling is the process and the result of creating a crosshatch pattern directly onto the shaft of the barbell. The purpose of this knurling is two-fold: to provide grip to the bar and serve as a guide (along with the rings) to help you place your hands consistently in the same place while performing various lifts.

For the most part, the placement of these markings conforms to either the International Powerlifting Federation (IPF) or IWF standards, although some bars include both markings.

Knurling in the center of the bar (center knurl) is designed to help keep the bar on your back when squatting and on your chest when performing front squats, thus most powerlifting bars include this. For bodybuilding, this center knurl is useful, because squats and front squats should form the core of your leg training. Additionally, many bars have smooth steel between knurls to protect the shins during deadlifts, cleans and snatches. Because good bodybuilders practice deadlifts, we like this too.

Knurling depth refers to how "sharp" the bar's crosshatch pattern feels in the hands and can range from passive to aggressive. This depth of knurling is a functional and personal preference. The deeper the knurl the more grip it will provide, but at the cost of tearing up the hands (calluses will form as your hands adapt). This is useful for many powerlifting movements such as deadlifts. Because bodybuilding uses a higher rep range than powerlifting, a deep knurl will quickly tear up the hands. I don't know too many women who work out that like to have the palms of their hands torn up or covered in calluses. For most bodybuilding exercises, a medium knurl will probably be best for most, which is what most barbell manufacturers provide. If you get a bar and find the knurling is too light, you can always use lifting chalk.

Finally, check out the length of the knurl. Because bodybuilding uses an expanded repertoire of movements, we often place our hands all over the bar, at vastly varying widths. Bars that have knurl that extend close to the sleeves allow us to have a secure grip at these varying widths.

Ring Spacing

This is the small, smooth-ringed areas between the knurling. Certified bars have standardized ring spacings so you can easily find your grip width on any standardized bar.

Plating & Finish

Many manufacturers add chrome, zinc, black oxide or other plating material (manganese phosphate, nickel) to their bars to prevent discoloration from oxidation and rust—it does not improve performance but makes an impact on maintenance. The location of your home gym can have a big effect on the maintenance of your bars and plates. Humid, damp environments invite oxidation and the formation of rust, so typical unfinished basements, sheds, and garages may require more metal maintenance than finished rooms and non-humid environments. If you're living in Nevada, Arizona or similar climates, then you can practically leave this stuff outside. In Maryland, we are notorious for having a confused climate, humid summers and spurts of extremely damp weather so rust is a common nuisance. In any case, pay attention to the plating and finish type of barbells in relation to your geographic and home gym location when obtaining these things.

For a home gym, the best bar coating options are the ones that provide the most rust protection and the least maintenance. That would be chrome (almost full rust resistance), zinc, and nickel-plated bars, followed by manganese phosphate. Trailing those, black oxide bars ooze the coolness factor, but like most cool things, come at a cost. (Technically, black oxide is not a coating but a treatment process that oxidizes the bar, providing only minimal rust resistance.) Uncoated bars (bare steel) provide no rust protection, require regular maintenance, but have a natural feel. There's just something good about gripping quality, natural steel.

So, why would you consider an uncoated or black oxide bar? Because adding a coating, plating or finish adds slickness to the bar, something that many lifters don't like and that may necessitate the use of lifting chalk at times, particularly with higher-rep hypertrophy work. The raw feeling of black oxide or bare steel is more conducive to low-rep, max effort lifts, where grip becomes much more significant of a factor.

In summary, here's what we want for a bodybuilding barbell.

A strong, straight bar that can handle loads up to 1000lbs with revolving 2" sleeves and center knurling. The depth of knurl and plating/finish are your preference.

Often, you can purchase a barbell and plate bundle for reduced cost. Just beware of inferior junk bars from mass-market retailers. Often, you're better off buying a good used bar secondhand.

If buying a used bar, pay particular attention to the tightness of the sleeve (it should not move from side-to-side or rattle), smoothness of the sleeve rotation (it should spin smoothly and quietly), and the straightness of the bar itself (roll it on the floor or on a rack—there should be no wobble).

Budget Barbell (less than $100)

I hesitate to even include this category here, because almost all new budget-based barbells are, shall we say kindly, *caveat emptor*. Or 'junk' to put it directly. Barbell coaches, such as Mark Rippetoe use stronger terms. The best bet here is a good quality used bar that someone is selling separately or with a pile of plates.

Economy Barbell ($100-$300)

This is where most of us will eventually land. Try to avoid mass-market bars and go with strong, durable bars from reputable companies such as York, Rogue Fitness and Texas Power Systems.

Luxury Barbell ($300+)

Of all the equipment items listed here, if you have the funds this is where to go luxury. That bar will be in your hands more than any other piece of fitness equipment over your lifetime (if you're training intelligently). Look for bars from Pendlay, Eleiko, Ivanko, Elite FTS, Werksan and York. Hard to go wrong from this bunch, especially around the $300 price point. (And yes, some bars actually do cost upwards of four figures, but for home gym bodybuilders, they are not necessary.)

Barbells vs. Dumbbells

Although dumbbells allow the aspiring bodybuilder to perform thousands of exercises and variations from seemingly unlimited angles, the barbell is the tool you'll use to pack on the majority of your muscle mass. Maneuvering a 300lb, loaded barbell is significantly easier than trying to handle two 150lb dumbbells. Likewise, getting set up for an exercise with an appropriate overload based on your level of progress and conditioning is far easier with a bar than with the bells. In that vein, besides the Olympic barbell, there are some specialty bars that the bodybuilder should have in their home gym arsenal.

Specialty Bars

Specialty bars can provide additional targeted tension and muscle isolation, something important to bodybuilders. Here are the specialty bars that have proven their effectiveness over time.

E-Z Curl Bar

First developed by Lewis G. Dymeck in the late 1940s, the E-Z Curl Bar is a short variant of the barbell designed to take some pressure off the wrists during curls. However, take a moment to think about the dual function of the biceps—to flex the elbow and supinate (turn up) the forearm/wrist. That latter function makes straight barbell curls, and especially dumbbell curls, so effective. They are maximizing both functions of the biceps. Alas, the E-Z Curl bar really fits it's name—it does make curling easier for the wrists (and easier in general)—at the expense of full supination. Therefore, suboptimal use of the biceps occurs. Is this what you want? Try curling the same weight with a barbell and then with an E-Z Curl bar. Notice which is *easier*. Remember, in hypertrophy training (bodybuilding), we want to make exercises harder (better).

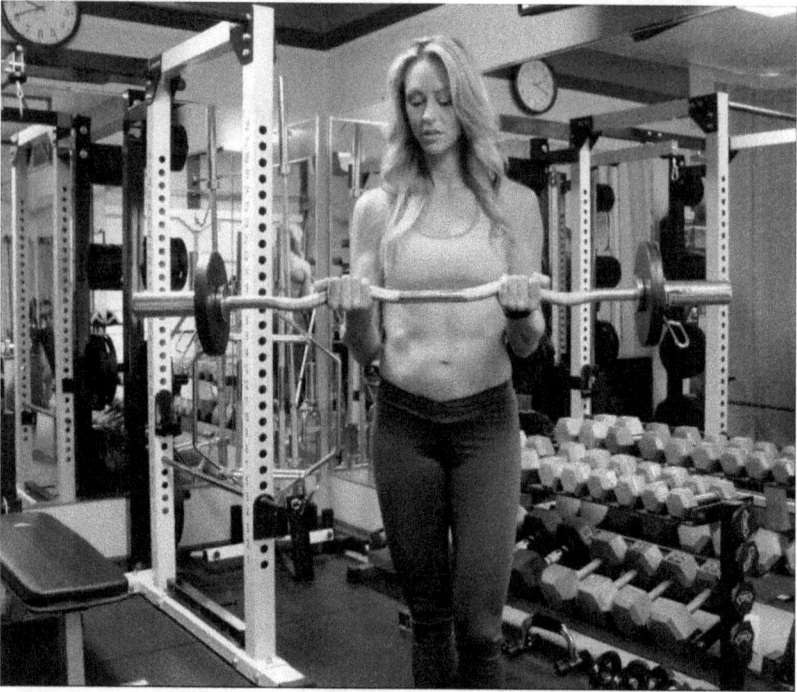

Where this bar really shines is with triceps work.

Many find that performing any type of triceps extension exercise is easier on the wrists and elbows with this bar, without affecting the stimulus to the triceps because we aren't changing or altering the function of that muscle group (extension of the elbow joint—straightening your arm).

E-Z Curl bars are plentiful in the used market. Make sure you get the Olympic variety and expect to spend about $30 to $80 bucks.

Triceps Bar

These short neutral-grip bars were originally designed to alleviate wrist or elbow issues for many triceps-centric exercises, such as extensions. However, they are also equally useful for hammer curls and some close-grip pressing, although you won't be able to use heavy loads here, due to the short bar length.

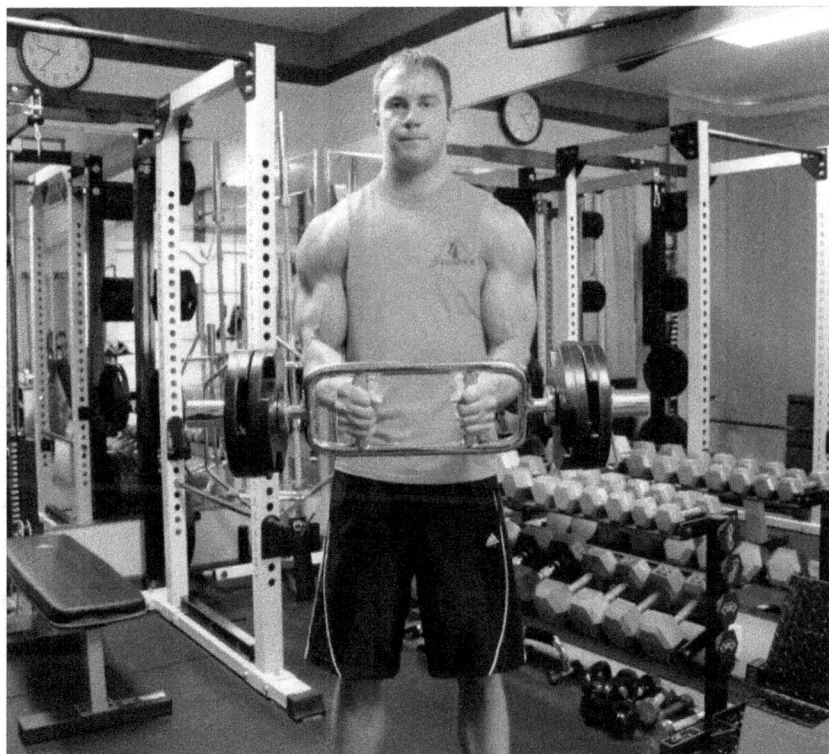

These bars cost anywhere from $30 to $90, and are readily available on the used market. Ensure you get the Olympic-sized variety with the rotating sleeves. For maximal loads with a neutral grip, the Multi-Grip bar is what you want.

Multi-Grip Bar (Swiss Bar)

This is an Olympic bar with several neutral handgrips in the center third of the bar, allowing you to perform barbell presses, rows and extensions with varying hand widths. The neutral grip is typically easier on the shoulders, because it does not place the shoulders into external rotation.

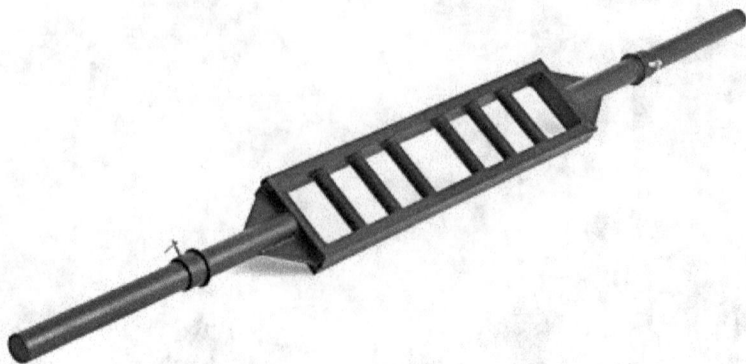

The downside here—these bars usually run about $300 and you'll probably have to buy a new one, because they are scarce in the used marketplace. I would only advise purchasing one of these after you have obtained an Olympic bar, E-Z Curl bar, triceps bar, and a trap bar. Unless you have pre-existing shoulder issues, in which case this bar may seem as if it came straight from the heavens.

Trap Bar (Hex Bar or Gerard Bar)

The hex (trapezius) bar, invented by powerlifter Al Gerard in the 1980s, is named for its unusual shape—it's a hexagonal Olympic barbell that allows you to perform various exercises from inside the encompassing bar.

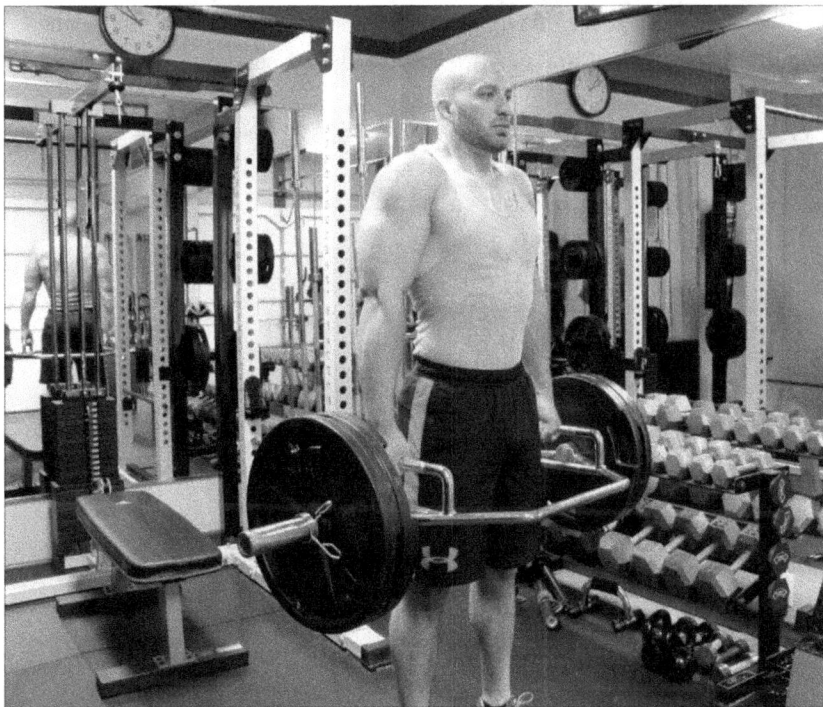

It's the shape and the corresponding way the load is balanced that makes this bar so useful (Mr. Gerard was trying to find a way to continue training with a chronic lower back injury). Due to the distribution of the weight in the center line of the body (unlike the barbell, which has the weight projected in front, or back of you), it assists the spine to maintain correct lumbar curvature when lifting weight from the floor. In simple terms, it places less compressive force on the spine. It also confers some additional benefits.

What is a Trap (Hex) Bar Good For?

Bigger, Stronger Trapezius Muscles

Let's start with the obvious. Other than picking up heavy barbell deadlifts and performing cleans, targeted trapezius training with trap bar shrugs is a damn effective method. The big problem with trap bar shrugging is that fairly soon you'll be able to shrug more weight than you can pick up off the floor. You can solve this by sitting on a small plyometric box located within the bar's center and performing the shrugs seated.

Increased Grip Strength

Allows for development of grip strength with less stress on the lower back.

Reduction of Lower Back Issues

Due to the positioning of your body *within* the center of the load.

Tall People

Exceptionally tall individuals with poor lever mechanics can safely pick up the load from the floor with this bar.

Variety of Movements

For neutral-grip presses, stride limitations on farmer's walks, etc. There's more…

What Else Can You Do With a Trap Bar?

So what can you do with it other than the obvious shrugging motion?

Here's a quick list:

- Deadlifts/Squats (it's great for deadlifts or for people who cannot safely perform regular deadlifts with a barbell, due to injury or lever disadvantages, such as especially tall individuals—if using the bar for squats, load up 25lb plates for a greater range of motion)
- Stiff Leg Deadlifts
- Upright Rows/High Pulls
- Farmer's Walk (prevents over-striding)
- Presses (a 'W' press, because you are able to bring your elbows lower than with a barbell)
- Push-ups (unloaded, it's a good alternative to those push-up handles)

- Ab rollouts (can substitute for an ab wheel, but with incremental loading and works the stabilizing muscles harder due to the increased difficulty of stabilization)

How Much is a Trap Bar Going to Cost?

At least $100. I've seen good, used trap bars at online and second-hand sporting goods stores for $100. Amazon sells them new for about $100-$150. High capacity (1000lbs), mega-trap bars, with longer sleeves that hold upwards of nine 45lb plates per side go for about $250. Most of us mere mortals won't need those, but their price offers us the high end of the expenditure scale.

5ft Olympic Barbell

Not many commercial gyms have these shorter five-foot Olympic bars, but they are maneuverable and work well in smaller spaces like most home gyms. You won't press, squat or deadlift with this bar, but it's great for curls, extensions and upright rows. I was able to a used one up at Play It Again Sports for $30. That's about the cost of a single container of protein powder, but will last far longer. Money well spent.

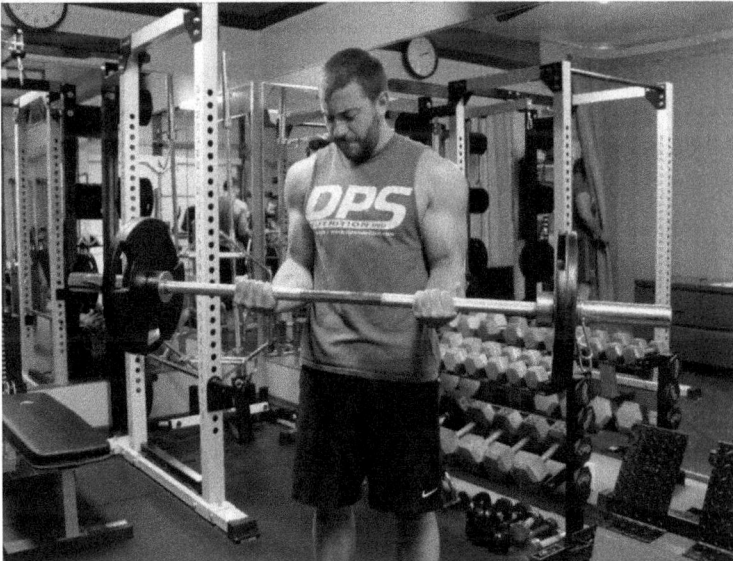

Cambered Barbell

My first gym had loads of Olympic bars, plates, benches and racks. And they had one strange barbell with the center portion bent to allow a greater range of motion when benching. At the time, I didn't know it was known as the McDonald Bar, named after the tremendous bench presser who trained with the bar to successfully increase his meet lift total.

The great secret to the bar's effectiveness is the increased range of motion permitted by the bar shape—allowing the elbows to retract further than with a barbell, offering the massive load capabilities and balance of the barbell, with the range of dumbbells. Thus, it's just as useful for rows as presses. Additionally, it's also effective for standing and seated shrugs, helping to reduce pressure on the lower back. In fact, at my first gym, seated shrugs with the cambered bar was probably the most popular movement with it. As far as I know, I was the only one there who used the bar for bent-over barbell rows—the effectiveness of those additional 1-2" of scapular retraction seemed to make a lot of difference to my growing back. And, well, we've already talked about the significance of an additional inch or two.

Since my original gym closed (a sad day, indeed) about twenty years ago, I've never seen a cambered barbell in any other gym I've visited. This is another chance to equip your home gym to greater heights than the commercial gyms. The problem will be locating one of these beasts. You can find them online, at specialty weightlifting stores. Expect to pay around $200 and don't spend you money on this type of bar until you already have all the others I've talked about previously. This bar is just icing on the cake.

One word of caution here—due to the extreme range of pressing motion with a cambered bar, the strain on the shoulder structure increases. Make sure you have the flexibility, connective tissue strength and are properly warmed up before using this type of bar. If in doubt, pass this one up for presses, but use it for rows and shrugs.

Fat Bars

Barbells with thick 2-2.5" shafts (fat bars) are exceptional for developing superior gripping strength and massive forearms because of the simple fact that they are harder to grip and hold onto as the load increases. Pick up and hold the same weight using an Olympic bar with a 1" shaft and then with a 2.5" shaft bar. I won't need to tell you which is more difficult. The weight did not increase, nor did the movement change. But your forearms will tell you which one is causing an adaptive response to occur.

Do you need to purchase specialized fat bars to get these benefits? Not anymore. With the advent of rubberized bar grips, you can turn just about any type of bar into a fat-grip version. More on this in the section on accessory equipment.

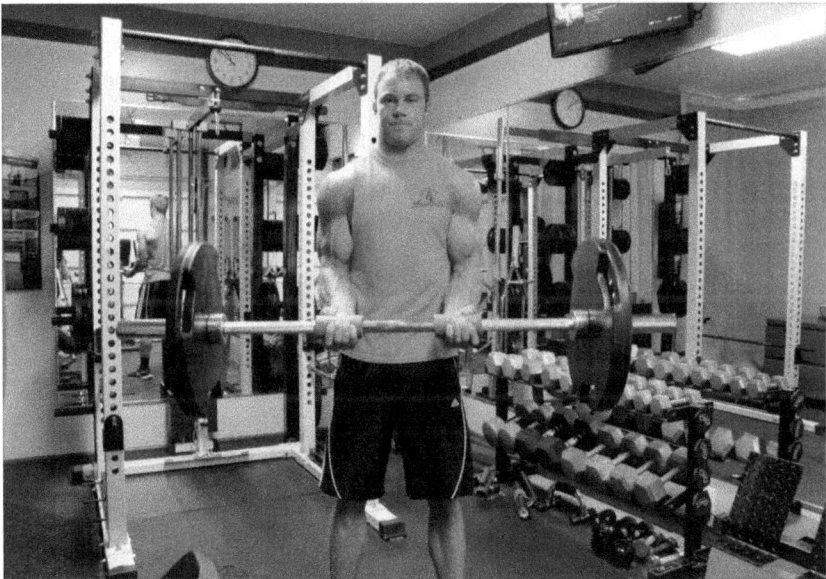

Budget Specialty Bars ($20-$120)
Beyond your barbell, the first stop should be a used E-Z Curl bar. Maneuverable in home gyms with plenty of versatility at low cost. After that, consider a trap bar due to its versatility.

Economy Specialty Bars ($140-$200)

Used or new E-Z Curl, Trap, and Triceps bars. That will provide you with maximum versatility on an economy budget.

Luxury Specialty Bars ($700+)

If you have a lot of funds (the Multi-Grip and Cambered bars are the expensive ones), there can never be enough bars in your home gym arsenal. Get the entire arsenal of specialty bars listed in this section. Your training partners will drool. If you don't have training partners in your home gym, these bars will attract some.

Bar Storage

Because your space is probably limited, bar racks are an efficient means to store a plethora of bars in a small amount of space. Bar gun racks are popular, but because the bars are stored horizontally, they occupy precious wall space that bodybuilders find essential (for mirrors!). Floor-based vertical bar holders are more practical for small spaces. I have a 9-bar floor-based bar rack tucked away in a corner of my home gym that occupies only two square feet—that's efficient storage per square foot.

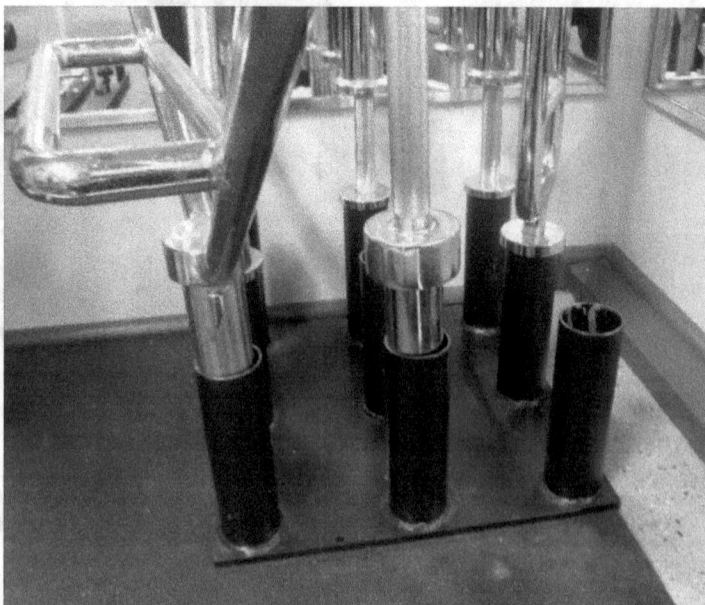

Because the typical bodybuilder will use several different bars (at least two, Olympic and E-Z Curl bars) I suggest building or obtaining a vertical bar storage solution.

DIY Bar Holder

Although commercial barbell holders cost anywhere from $50-$150 (used and new), you can make one quickly for about ten bucks. Here's how.

You'll need a cinder block, some 2" PVC pipe and concrete. Set the cinder block on a sheet of scrap plywood, cut the PVC a couple inches longer than the height of the block, insert the PVC into the holes and pour the concrete into the gaps between the pipe and the block. Done. Each of these cinder block bar holders can accommodate eight Olympic-size bars. The equivalent commercial bar holder would cost you over $100. Spray paint the block black or whatever color suits you for the "finishing" touch.

You can also use this DIY project to hold brooms, shovels or any other long implements. Just use appropriate diameter PVC for these modifications.

Budget Barbell Storage ($10)

Take the DIY route and be done in about ten minutes for ten bucks. Holds eight bars.

Economy Barbell Storage ($50-$75)

Because you probably won't need or even have upwards of eight bars, buy a used (or new) bar holder that accommodates six bars (standard bar, 5' bar, E-Z Curl, Triceps bar, Trap bar). Because this is not lifting equipment, going the used route is preferable, if the price is right.

Luxury Barbell Storage ($100+)

For the bar masochists out there (me!), cut to the chase and get a bar holder that accommodates 9-12 bars. That's what I needed, because I have two rack-based stations, multiple training partners and use lots of bars.

Collars & Clamps

In any athletic endeavor, taking safety precautions is paramount. Weightlifting, like any other athletic movement, can be an inherently dangerous activity. Making sure our plates don't fall off our bars and dumbbell handles is the least we can do here.

You want something that is easy to take on and off the bar, while ensuring a tight hold. There are several options, including spring clamps, ratchet clamps, and bolt on collars. Each has advantages and disadvantages.

Spring Clamps

These are cheap and effective for bar use, but due to their size, don't work as well with dumbbell handles.

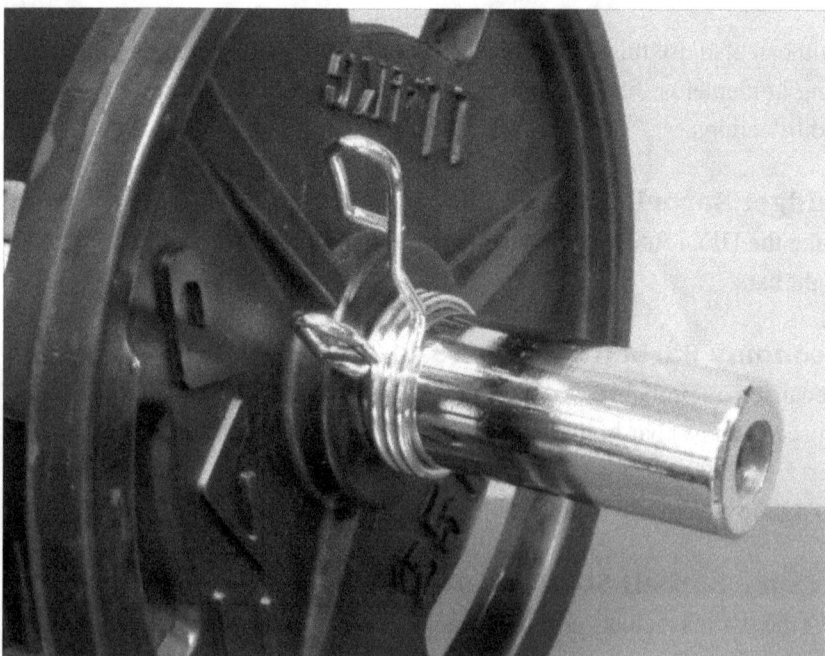

Additionally, over time, the spring can become loose—something we definitely don't want, especially with a dumbbell exercise where the bell is over your head (pullovers, presses and extensions). Spring clamps are cheap (about a dollar or two) and quick to attach/remove, but offer the least amount of reliability.

Ratchet Clamps

These are heavy duty, single-action cam locks that securely clamp the collar to the bar. Lock-Jaw clamps are the most popular type in this category. They attach/remove quickly and provide high reliability. They won't come off during your set.

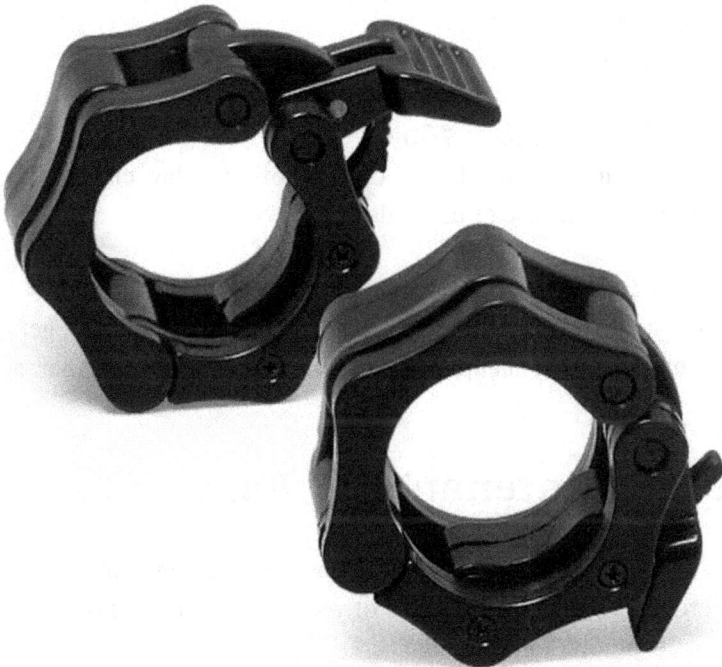

However, they are quite expensive, compared to the simple spring clamps. Additionally, an average pair of ratchet-type clamps occupies about two inches of the bar's sleeve length and adds about a pound to the bar load—a trivial amount for some, but something to factor in for advanced trainers.

Bolt-On Collars

All you need to know here are that bolt-on collars require a wrench to tighten and loosen them for bar attachment and removal. This is a big time-wasting nuisance to the home gym lifter—something that can quickly dampen the best training enthusiasm. Additionally, they offer no safety advantages over spring collars or ratchet clamps, so it's best to avoid them.

The bottom line here is make sure the barbell collars you use are up for the task. Because we have such a variety of tasks in bodybuilding training, you may want to have several types of collars on-hand.

Budget Collars ($5-$10)
Use spring clamps, because they are cheap and effective.

Economy Collars ($20-$60)
Get yourself a pair of spring clamps and a set of Lock-Jaw clamps. The best of both worlds in ease of use and security.

Luxury Collars ($100+)
If you've gone the luxury route for bars, then you have many. So, get yourself a pair of spring clamps and Lock-Jaws for each type of bar, as warranted.

Care & Maintenance of Bars

Like any piece of finely machined steel, bars require some upkeep. If you provide proper care and maintenance of your barbells, they should remain in excellent condition for a lifetime.

We are concerned about the general upkeep of the bar, as well as the rotational (functional) aspects.

Occasional brushing with a steel brush eliminates dead skin cells from the knurling as well as removing any minor rust buildup. At my local Gold's Gym, they haven't used a brush to clean the dead skin remnants from any of the barbells—ever. That's over ten years of other people's DNA there, which is occasionally useful for getting sick.

Apply WD-40 to the internal bushing or bearing area, where the sleeve meets the bar. Work the oil into the area (place a 25lb plate on the sleeve and spin the plate) and wipe clean. Apply a generous amount of oil to the end of the bar, through the hole in the cap. Tip the bar up so the oil runs down the bar into the inside bearing/bushing assembly. Let the bar stand for a couple hours. Then, wipe off any excess oil and do the other end the same way.

Add regular bar upkeep to your overall home gym maintenance checklist. I'll talk more about this at the end of the equipment section.

Racks—Lifting to the Limit, Safely

Eventually, you are going to get too strong for dumbbell use exclusively. Dumbbell deadlifts will no longer be a challenge. Goblet squats will tax your upper body more so than your legs. The barbell becomes essential for adaptation to continue.

One of the disadvantages to training at home is the lack of spotters when handling heavy weights on the bar. Enter the power rack.

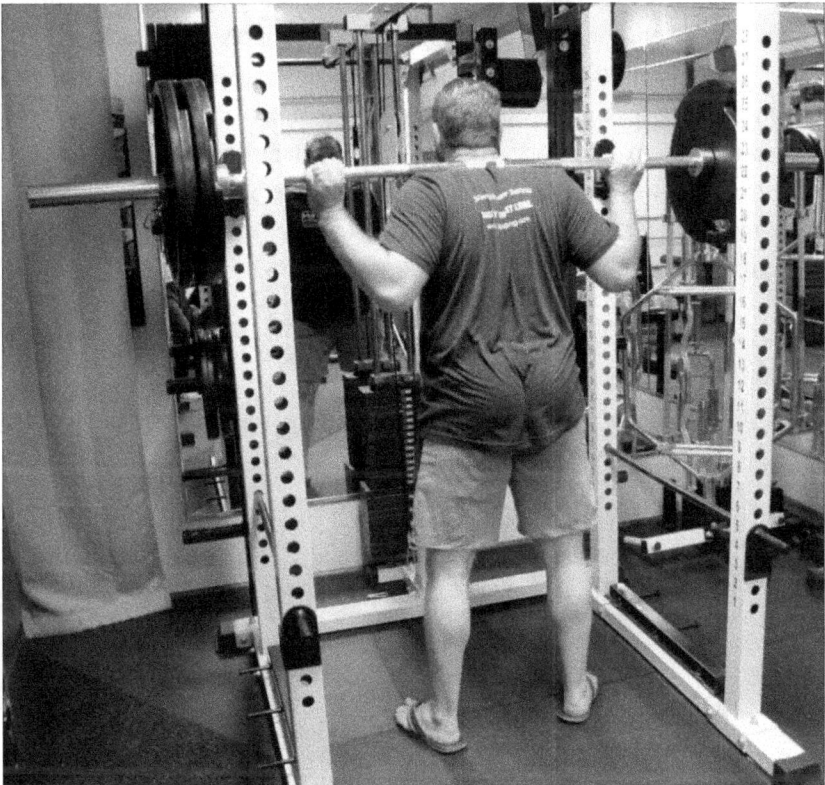

Power racks facilitate getting the barbell into position for things like squats and presses and are the safest way to lift big weights. They are fully enclosed beasts that have adjustable safety bars, which when set up properly act as your spotters and will catch any weight that you drop. Most of us subconsciously hold back on many lifts, such as squats and presses, for fear of failing with the weight at that last crucial, transformative rep, or for fear of injury. With a power rack, you can perform bench presses in there and won't get pinned under the bar or drop it on your head. You can squat without fear of not being able to stand up again. You can actually train with true intensity with a barbell in solitude. This is how to train at home.

Power racks allow us to lift heavy weights with minimal equipment—safely.

Power racks form the centerpiece of our bodybuilding gym. They are not optional. You won't be able to lift a barbell in a progressively heavier manner safely without one. They allow us to train in safety with basic, compound exercises that form the bedrock of adaptive change. Every other isolation exercise we are concerned with here emanates outside of this centrifuge. A power cage coupled with an Olympic barbell forms the perfect marriage—a lifetime of adventure, struggle, glorious success and disappointing setbacks.

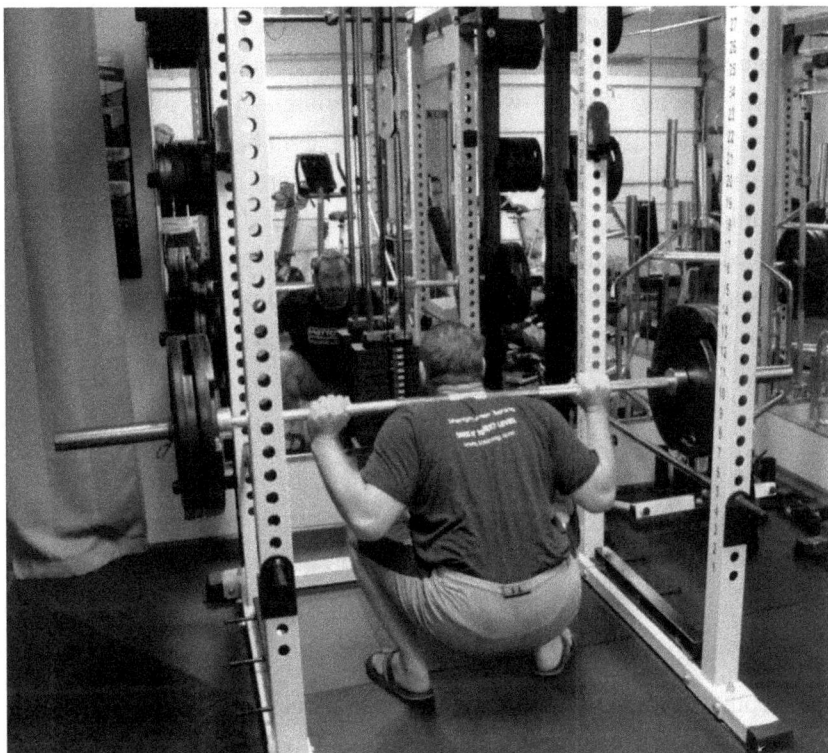

Modern power racks are like the Erector™ sets of the weightlifting world. Beyond the various heights, widths and cage depth, there are a seemingly endless list of features, accessories and possibilities. For many, especially those of us with limited funds and critical thought to not wasting money, it can be daunting to determine just which rack best fits our location, concerns and resources. So, let's look at the variables you need to consider when selecting a power rack for home gym bodybuilding.

Foremost, is the rack's footprint—how much room is this thing going to occupy. The combination of height, width, and depth determine the power rack's frame size and what you can do in there.

Height

This is where your ceiling height comes into the equation. It's also where the ability to perform standing presses becomes important. If your ceiling can't accommodate the rack height, then you need to find a shorter rack (shorter racks also cost less). Also, consider if you will ever move your gym from the current location to another locale. For example, although my home gym is in my garage—with nine foot ceilings—I was aware that sometime in the future I may need to move the gym back into my basement—which only has eight foot ceilings. Therefore, I opted for a rack that would fit in both locations. Finally, consider head clearance space over and above the height of the rack for standing presses and chinning exercises as well. If the rack doesn't allow for standing presses, you'll need to use the less effective seated version of the exercise for maximum safety.

Width

Next, look at rack width. Most racks are standard in width, because the Olympic barbell length largely dictates cage width. Remember, you need to move to the sides of the rack to load the bar.

Depth

Rack depth determines how much forward and backward space you have for bar travel. For powerlifting, rack depth is not as crucial, because the bar travels in a straight line for squats, presses and deadlifts. However, to accommodate the expanded world of bodybuilding exercises with arc-based movements, such as curls and extensions, we need a rack with greater depth. Look for power racks with depths of at least 24". In excess of thirty inches is even better. Cheaper racks have narrow depth, so deeper racks will add to the cost.

The combination of rack height, width and depth determines the caged environment you'll live in for many of your most transformational movements, so make sure you can live with it once the choice has been made. You're going to spend a lot of time in there.

Open or Closed Top

Most power racks have a closed top. This increases the stability of the rack and typically provides space for an attached chinning bar. Open racks allow you to perform standing presses and other overhead exercises.

Because we ultimately want a rack that includes options for a chinning bar and a cable pulley system, open racks are not what we want.

Stabilizer Bar

Some racks include a stabilizer frame bar that runs along the lower back of the rack, keeping the rack stable, if not anchored to the floor. You don't want a rack with this bar. It presents nothing but a hindrance to your feet when un-racking the barbell for a squat or pressing movement. It also impedes certain placements of your adjustable bench. Avoid.

Capacity

These things should be able to handle close to 1,000lbs on the spotter rails/rods. Over time, you'll be surprised how strong you can get. If the rack you're interested in doesn't specifically list the weight capacity, look for another rack.

Frame Gauge

The industry standard frame gauge for a power rack is 2"x3" 11-gauge steel. Anything less will have a lower weight capacity and stability, whereas higher gauges are just like riding around in an Abrams M1 tank— awesome, if you can afford them.

Weight

In general, the weight of an empty rack provides a big clue to the stability and overall ruggedness of the thing. Wide, deep and tall racks with large frame gauges will weigh the most. Cheap racks made of cheap steel only weigh about 150-200lbs. If your life is going to depend on the stability and capacity of the rack, then I think you'll want a heavy beast.

Hole Pattern & Spacing

Hole spacing is measured in the distance from the center of two adjacent holes on the uprights. This distance affects your reach, level of comfort and range of motion when setting up and performing exercises. For example, an inch or two may not make a difference when setting up for a squat, but can have a huge difference in pressing. Additionally, this spacing may end up being a critical aspect in your ability to progress past training plateaus.

Good racks don't exceed a 2" spacing. Great racks use a 1-1.5" Westside Barbell (Louie Simmons) spacing scheme, especially within the deadlift, bench and clean/pull-up areas. Typically, the closer the hole spacing, the higher the quality of the overall rack—and thus the higher the price.

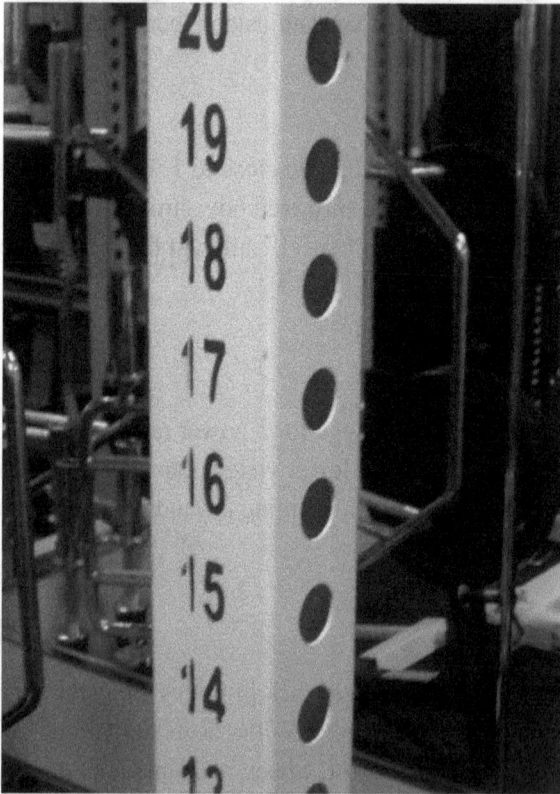

If the rack you are investigating only has the industry standard 2" spacing, you can still slide a 1" piece of plywood or series of rubber horse stall mat pieces under your bench (or feet for deadlifts) to achieve those 1" increments. That's a tip right from Mr. Simmons himself.

Numbered Posts

Racks with 2" hole spacing (or less) have lots of holes—the good kind. It really helps if those holes come pre-numbered so you can quickly adjust the safety rods and write that type of info in your training logs. Believe me, as you change exercises, constantly counting for the correct hole on each upright becomes a pain in the gluteus. If the rack you're looking at doesn't have numbered posts, this is not a deal killer. You can always write them on with a permanent marker or some paint.

Rods vs. Rails

Besides the frame itself, the secondary safety aspect of power racks is the safety pins, rods or rails that can be set at multiple heights using the hole posts. These safety accoutrements catch the bar if you miss a lift. In the preference battle between rods versus rails, two elements emerge—speed of adjustments and exercise impact.

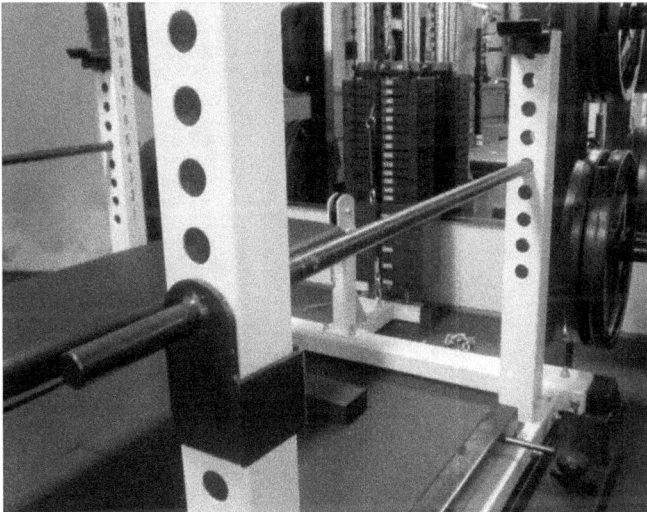

Typically, rods are the fastest to adjust. Modern rail-based systems should have pop-pins for quick and easy height changes. As for exercise impact, here's what I'm talking about. Some training techniques, such as touch-and-go and pin pressing, require repeated touching of the bar to the safety rods/rails. Many times, the bar does not contact these rods/rails at both ends simultaneously as you perform a rep. For rounded rods, this is not a problem—your movement pattern does not change by contact with the rod. However, some rail-based systems, particularly those that do not lock but instead hang from adjustment hooks, will start swinging as the bar contacts them. This is not good. On your next contact of the barbell to the rail, this can often disrupt your movement pattern and create an unsafe situation for your connective tissue and other dearly held soft tissue.

So, my preference is always for rod-based power racks. They were the first, and still the best. Sometimes, modernization does not produce improvements.

J-Hooks

These are the hooks where you rack the bar. The important consideration here is that they not be too deep, otherwise it becomes hazardous when taking the bar out for a lift. Additionally, if they are too shallow—well, you can imagine what happens there. We want hooks that allow you to easily lift the bar out and not up. Lifting the bar up compromises starting execution and setup.

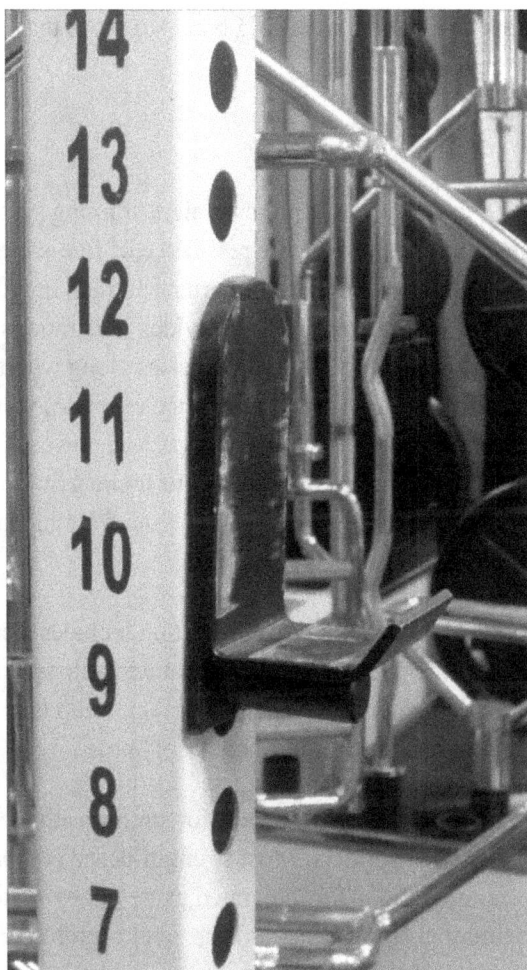

Finally, realize that there is interplay here between hole spacing and J-Hook design. Closer hole spacing greatly alleviates issues with J-Hooks.

Pull-Up Bar

Integrated pull-up bars, attached to a power rack, adds the entire world of chinning exercises to your training repertoire. Although you can easily make a decent pull-up bar with plumbing pipe and fittings, we really want the chinning bar incorporated into the power rack for maximum exercise flexibility and space savings. Look for bars that are completely straight, have appropriate knurling and give a big bonus to those that incorporate neutral-grips in the design.

Cable Pulley System

Invented in the 19th century, cable pulley weight-training systems provide constant resistance, unlike the variable resistance of free-weight exercises. To the aspiring bodybuilder, both are important. In fact, in Bill Pearl's excellent *Keys to the Inner Universe*, he provides illustrations and descriptions of hundreds of cable-based exercises along with the free weight stuff. There are some constant resistance exercises you just can't duplicate with free weights—things like triceps pushdowns and side lateral raises. So, having a cable pulley system in your home gym opens up additional portions of the exercise universe to your training and provides a different type of resistance.

You have two options here: get a power rack that includes a cable pulley system at the back of the rack, or obtain a separate cable apparatus, such as a lat pull-down/seated row combo. The power rack setup is preferred, because that occupies almost no additional floor space.

This is where traditional power racks built for strength athletes differ from those more useful to bodybuilders. Most strength-based companies only sell racks that offer no options for integrated cable pulley systems. For bodybuilders, training in home gyms, this presents a problem.

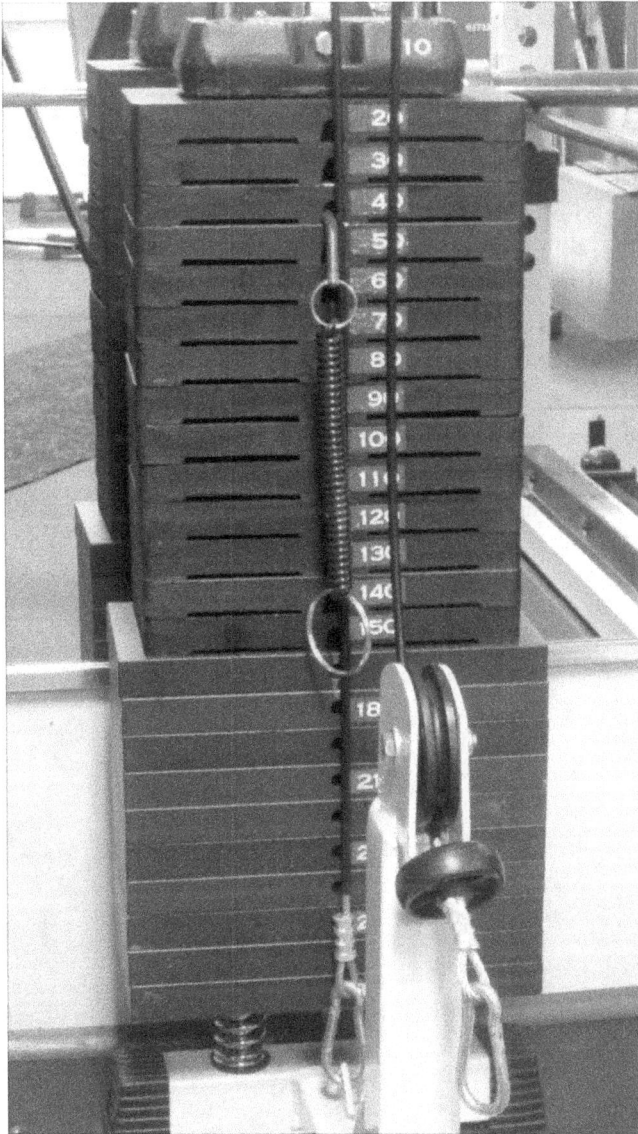

My strong recommendation, especially those with tight training quarters, is to obtain a power rack with an integrated cable pulley system or at least the option to add one when you have the means. There are two types here: the more common and less expensive plate-loaded variety and the weight stack version. Although your budget may dictate which you choose, at least consider that weight stack versions offer the ability to change the weight rapidly, simply by removing and inserting a pin at the appropriate weight setting in the stack. For techniques such as drop sets or Russian ladders, this becomes important and eliminates the drudgery of constantly adding and removing plates from the back pulley's carriage.

Dip Handles

As John McCallum so astutely noted throughout his landmark book, *Keys to Progress*, dips are one of the most important and adaptation inducing exercises available. Many refer to them as squats for the upper body, so that should put them in perspective.

You have two options for including dipping bars in your home gym. Mount a set to the wall (not likely if you rent or have limited space) or obtain a set of dip handles that attach to your power rack. I think you're starting to see how integral the power rack is to training.

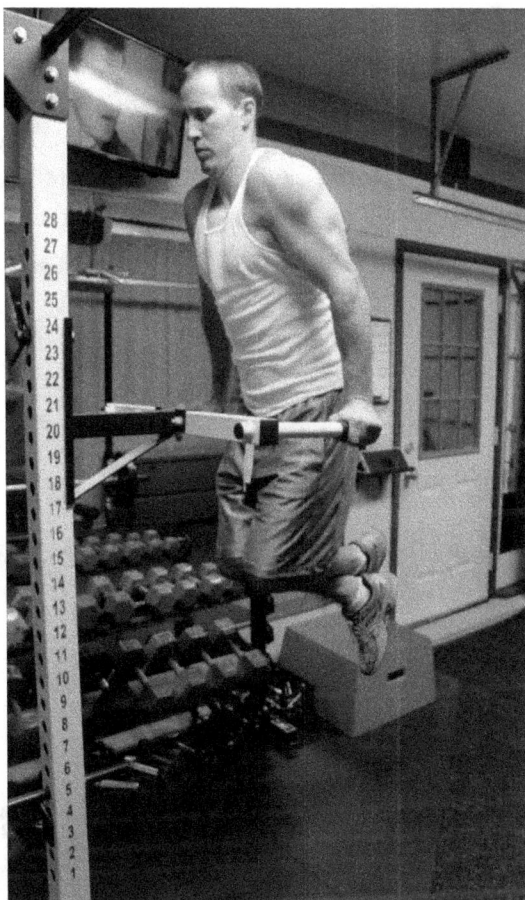

In either case, take note of the width between dip handles and their direction. For optimal comfort and effectiveness, dip handles should be spaced approximately 22" apart and have an outward angle, allowing you to adjust your grip width by moving closer or farther from the ends of the handles. Additionally, note the handle diameter. You don't want handles that are smaller than your bar diameter. Larger diameter handles are good for additional grip and triceps work, but you can always add rubberized handle clamps, so don't worry about this too much—just be sure the handles are not smaller than your barbell's shaft diameter. That can cause issues such as forearm pain.

Plate Storage

Although we've already looked at plate storage earlier, it's important to note that some racks offer integrated plate storage, so this might be an important consideration for space saving. It's also the option I choose for my garage gym and I can tell you it both keeps the weights out of the way, off the floor and easily accessible to the bar on the rack.

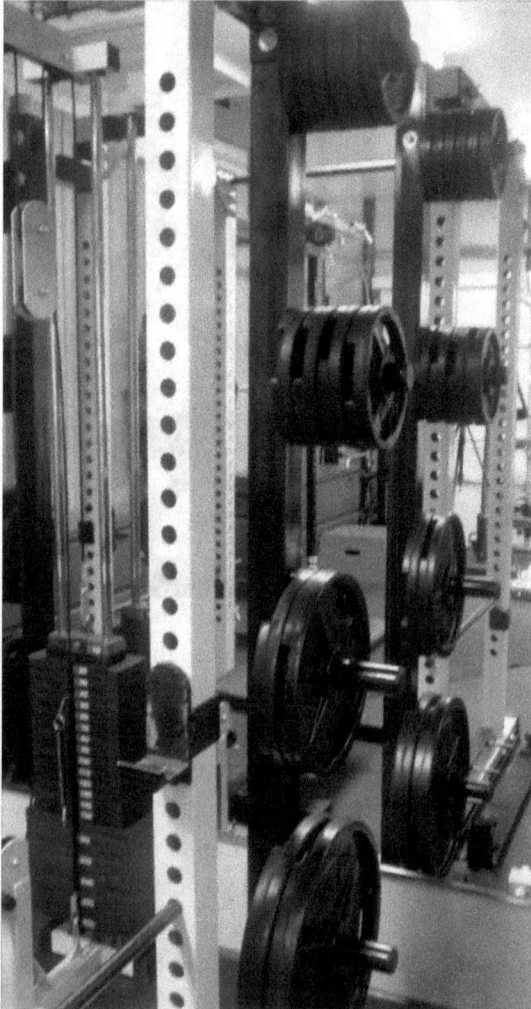

Bar Storage

Some racks do offer integrated bar storage but that's exactly what they offer—storage for one, or at most, two bars. We need more than that, so use one of the external bar storage options discussed earlier and don't worry about integrated bar storage on the rack. If it has it, fine. If not, we don't care.

Band Pegs

One last consideration is band pegs. What are they? Although familiar to strength lifters, most bodybuilders have never used them. Band pegs are simply externally facing pegs or posts located at the bottom (and sometimes top) of the rack used to secure the end of rubberized resistance bands to the rack and the other end to your barbell. This provides enhanced variable resistance to free weight exercises—much like chains—to barbell work. It's particularly useful for improving strength in presses and squats, both from the start and lockout.

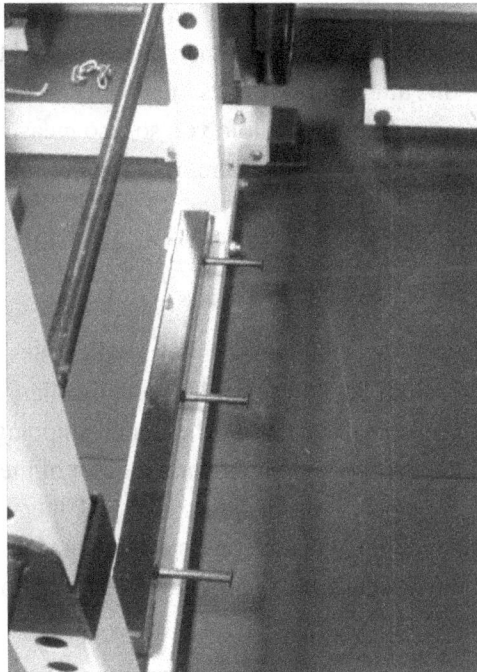

Because band training is not particularly central to hypertrophy training, the inclusion or omission of band pegs on your power rack will not impact your results.

Compatibility with Accessories from Other Manufacturers

Eventually, you may want additional rods, J-Hooks, plate storage, etc. Power racks with industry standard frame sizes/gauges are typically compatible with accessories like this across different manufacturers, thus increasing your options and usually decreasing cost to you.

Color Options

Does it really matter? This should be the least of your concerns.

Assembly & Transport

Most power racks bolt together from separate pieces—a few come pre-welded, except for cross members. Make sure you can get the rack or the rack pieces through any doors, halls, corners, etc. required to place it in its new home. Often, this afterthought elicits the mighty, "well damn", among other things—and now I can say, "I told you so", so measure *everything* before you obtain it. That's a good general rule for any substantial piece of exercise equipment or life furnishings.

Cost (including shipping)

Power racks are heavy, even the inexpensive, smaller ones. You can end up paying anywhere from $250 to several thousand dollars for new racks. Often, due to the weight of these things, the freight shipping costs will be in the hundreds, sometimes adding up to half the cost of the rack itself. One way to eliminate much of that expense is to pick them up direct from a warehouse, if feasible. Some manufacturers even ship racks free (hint: especially around the holidays and New Years)—so look for that.

Brands

Good power rack brands come from the likes of York, EliteFTS, Texas Strength Systems, PowerTec, and BodyCraft.

To recap, in this section I presented you with a list of variables to consider when thinking about getting a rack. There's a lot of things to think about. My suggestion is to make a spreadsheet or at least write down what each power rack offers that you are considering so that you can easily compare your options. The choice that most closely meets your needs, location and budget should quickly jump out to you from that comparison.

For those truly dedicated and capable (or lacking funds), you can always build your own power rack.

DIY Power Rack

Because power racks are affordable (especially used racks), I do not generally advise building one from wood or pipe, unless you have no room for a rack indoors and must place it outside for year-round use. That's where pressure-treated and stained wood power racks shine. However, if you are an able welder with access to metal fabricating machinery, then go for it. I have one lifting acquaintance who built his that way, and it turned out to be a damn fine beast.

You can make safe and effective power racks out of wood or steel. Wood? Really? Yes, actually. What's your house or apartment made of? Lots of wood nailed or screwed together in an intelligently engineered solution—which holds lots of load too. Therefore, you welders out there should opt for the metal DIY plans and the carpenters can choose a wood-based plan. Some of the wood-based plans allow you to construct a rack for under $100. Of course, your time is also money.

Strength coach extraordinaire, Mark Rippetoe, provides one of the most complete sets of plans for building your own power rack, providing the detailed design schematic for sizing, cutting and welding the steel for the job—however, note that his plans are for a shallow, strength training rack with no affordance for a cable-pulley system. If you do an Internet search for "DIY power rack", many more good designs (and some bad ones) are available, with and without cables.

Power Rack vs. Smith Machine

Some of you may be tempted to forgo the traditional power rack in lieu of the more glamorous Smith machine. Unless you already own a power rack, I urge you to resist this siren song. At the surface, it may seem that the Smith machine offers the same benefits as the power rack—versatility, safety and confidence—but it comes at a cost. Smith machines don't improve your balance, stability and coordination—and they don't activate stabilizer muscles. They are great for muscle isolation and for working through or around injuries— which is why I do recommend them as a luxury item for advanced bodybuilders who already have all the basic equipment.

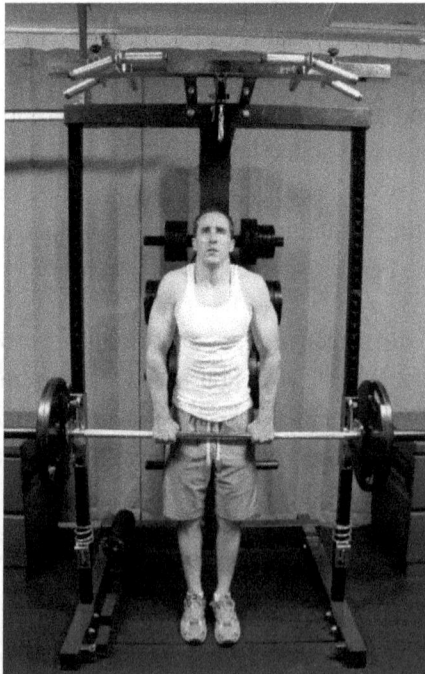

For those advanced bodybuilders who have well-developed stabilizers and already own a power rack and can afford the cost and space in the home gym, a Smith machine affords the ability to challenge the prime movers *by*

increasing stability. It also helps to spare the nervous system in advanced lifters who may be teetering on the over-reaching, over-training precipice. Again—Smith machines are not useful for novice, or even intermediate bodybuilders, but can provide an infrequent and valuable tool for the advanced. I am not ashamed to admit that I have a Smith machine in my home gym, right next to the power rack.

Racks and Stands You Don't Want

I want to take a minute and talk about a couple pieces of equipment that you might be tempted to purchase, due to their lower price point, but that I don't recommend primarily from safety and versatility standpoints. Let's start from the least expensive and versatile.

Squat Stands

These things are great if you're an experienced powerlifter, or are always lifting with other experienced trainers—in home gyms, the latter is not likely. Squat stands don't take up much space and are really good for loading up a bar and having it at chest level for presses and squats.

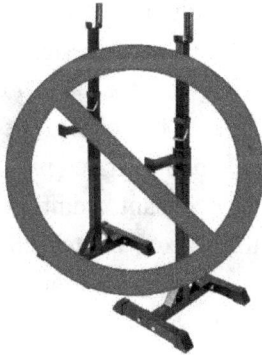

However, they provide zero safety if you fail on those presses and squats—thus the need for other, experienced lifters. Because I'm assuming you are lifting at home, alone—these are no good for you. Please don't fool yourself here.

Squat Rack

These are dedicated racks in most commercial gyms and are useful for squats, presses and loading bars for shrugs, and—god forbid—curling.

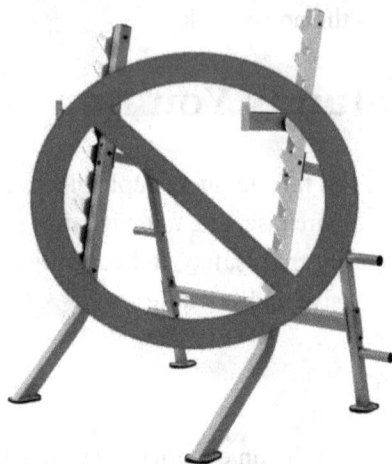

A step up from squat stands in safety, they may include plate storage at the rear of the rack, which does offer another attraction from a home gym perspective. More expensive than squat stands but cheaper than half and full rack systems, there are two big problems for the home gym lifter here—versatility and safety. Squat racks designed for squatting—although you can use the various spotting pins for loading the bar for overhead pressing and the fixed spotter rails for loading the bar for shrugs (and those curls)—that's about it. There's no integrated pull-up bar, so that's going to be another expense and space occupant. Additionally, if you are exceptionally short or tall, those fixed spotter rails may not be in the most optimal place for you in terms of range of motion or safety. Squat racks do provide some safety—as long as you don't fall or lose your balance backward when squatting or pressing. Again, not a great choice for working out alone and therefore, not recommended.

Half Racks

I'm not a big fan of half racks for one main reason—safety. They share the same issue as squat stands, in that they provide no recourse if you fail backwards in a lift. And although they best squat racks by having an adjustable rail system (typically via monster J-hooks), half racks provide half the functionality of a power rack within the same amount of space— and they typically don't allow you to add things like dipping bars. Right there, that should end the discussion.

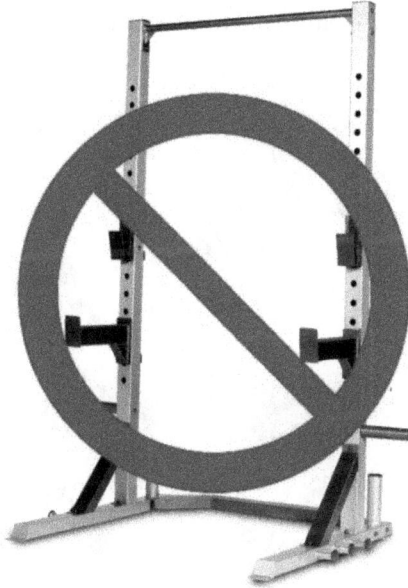

Budget Racks ($250-$500)

You can easily find budget-based power racks on Internet retailer sites and second-hand markets with prices ranging from $250-$500. Just realize that with this low price comes some others things. Make sure you review the specs against the various attributes listed above to make sure the rack will work for you. And yes, you can build yourself a rack for less than $250— but make sure you follow a solid and reputable engineering plan here and test the thing before you get in it.

Economy Racks ($500-$1000)

If you can afford a rack in this price range, I highly suggest making the investment. Racks here will usually meet all of the demanding criteria listed above. They are generally sturdier and safer with heavy loads than the budget racks.

Luxury Racks ($1000+)

For most, an reputable economy rack will suffice. For those who want 3" steel tubing, modular rack systems, extreme height for standing presses and the ability to load your car on the thing, then yes, racks in the four figure range are available. You won't need to concern yourself about safety or stability here.

Machines—What is Really Necessary?

Aside from the dumbbells, barbells, plates, bench and rack, there are a few additional essential pieces of equipment that a bodybuilder will need. I say 'essential', although early bodybuilding legends such as John Grimek and Steve Stanko didn't have access to some of this stuff—because it wasn't invented yet or commonplace in most gyms. Believe me, if they had access to this equipment, they would have used it.

Because muscle isolation and necessity is the bodybuilder's mother of invention, equipment that provided loading and enhanced time under tension for lat pulldowns, triceps pushdowns, leg extensions, leg curls, and seated calf raises were born. And if you look, the subsequent improvements in bodybuilder's back, triceps, and leg development over the course of those machine inventions, most notably in shape and separation became evident. Therefore, these machines are our new normal, our modern day essentials that afford maximum isolation training that would be difficult to perform with barbells or dumbbells.

Right away, you'll notice that legs are the big consideration here so let's start there.

Leg Extensions & Leg Curls

As mentioned, bodybuilders of the 1940s and 1950s had no leg isolation machinery for the quadriceps and hamstrings—only iron boots. If you don't know what they are, consider yourself blessed to be living in modern times.

Most leg isolation machines—particularly the leg extension and leg curl—can be traced back to the late 1940s inventions by George Redpath and Jack Lalanne. Today, you can easily outfit your home bodybuilding gym with a leg curl and leg extension device. But, there are a few things to consider here.

Capacity

Because you will be isolating your quadriceps and hamstrings with leg extensions and curls, obviously you won't be able to handle the same poundages there as with squats and stiff-leg deadlifts. However, you still need to ensure that the leg extension and curl apparatus you obtain can handle sufficient loads to provide adaptive stress in an isolated environment. I've seen many advanced trainers work up to and beyond two hundred pounds in these movements, so don't sell yourself short if you are just starting out and note the capacity of the apparatus before making a decision.

Range of Motion

Make sure the range of motion on the leg extension and curl doesn't sell you short of your natural range either. Because you only develop strength in the range of motion trained (with some radiating effects), you don't want to be limited to a significant subset of your inherent range. Although commercial weight-stack leg machines provide a generous range, many plate-loaded varieties do not. Check this before buying.

Comfort

You don't want your shins to hate you, so make sure the pads on the leg extension device are ample under heavy load. That means we want thick and dense foam here.

With capacity, range of motion, and comfort considerations firmly in mind, you now have three basic types of leg extension/curl apparatus to ponder.

Plate-Loaded Leg Extension/Curl Attachment

These attach to your adjustable bench and accept barbell plates to vary the resistance. Most accept standard size plates with 1" diameter holes, so you will need to acquire an Olympic plate adaptor to fit onto the weight yoke here.

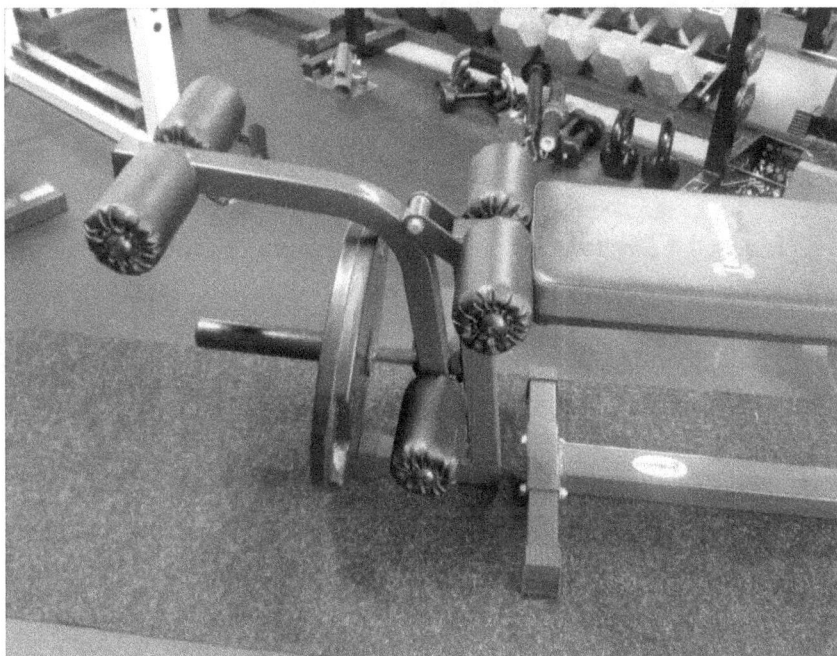

Using an attachment for your leg extension and curl movements saves both money and space—however, the amount of plate resistance that can be added (capacity) will tend to be limited here.

Standalone Plate-Loaded Leg Extension/Curl

Taking the plate-loaded route one-step further, standalone leg extension/curl machines offer a more commercial gym experience, but keep the cost down by combining the two movements into a single machine, and by employing the plate-loaded model. Standalone units can handle more weight than the attachment version, because they do not rely on a single point of attachment for stability.

However, they take up precious home gym real estate, especially if you opt for dedicated units specifically designed for leg extensions and lying leg curls.

Standalone Stack-Based Leg Extension/Curl

The penultimate method to isolate and overload your quadriceps and hamstrings is to obtain dedicated standalone machine-stack based leg extension and curl machines. Just like commercial gyms.

If you have the means to go this route (and it's an expensive purchase for isolating the front and back of your thighs), you'll find your best options by scouring the Internet for older, used units or snagging ones from gym closings or gyms undergoing equipment upgrades. (Earlier, I mentioned my epic fail to jump on the used Cybex leg machines deal for $300 each. Don't follow my lead there.) If you buy one of these things new, you might as well just open your own gym, because new leg isolation machines can start at $3000. In any case, these things take up lots of space.

Budget Leg Extension/Curl ($50-$100)
There's only one budget choice here—a plate-loaded leg extension/curl attachment. Remember, you might need an Olympic sleeve adaptor to fit your plates on securely.

Economy Leg Extension/Curl ($350-$500)
A standalone, plate-loaded combination extension./curl machine is your friend here. You've already got the plates and this will take up half the space of separate units. If your legs are exceptionally strong, standalone units allow you to load much more than their attachment-based counterparts.

Luxury Leg Extension/Curl ($600-$6000)
Separate, standalone, weight-stack based machines (you need one for extensions and another for curls). Scan for used units—otherwise, your bank account and floor space are going to take a big hit.

Seated Calf Raise

Due to the anatomical construction of the calves, you need to perform calf raises in two positions—with your legs straight and bent (seated). Seated calf raises fully isolates and activates the soleus muscle, which give the calves that diamond shape when viewed from the front or back. For serious bodybuilders, this is (or should be!) serious work.

Before the invention of the dedicated seated calf raise machine by George Redpath in 1949 (a busy year for the guy—thanks George!), bodybuilders resorted to placing a heavy barbell across their thighs while seated.

You can still do the same, although it's not easy or comfortable as the load increases. For advanced trainers, you'll want some type of seated calf raise apparatus. As with most leg-based machinery, you'll want to consider these things:

Ease of Use

There's a reason good old George Redpath invented the seated calf raise machine. It's not easy, especially as you get stronger, to hoist a heavy barbell or dumbbell onto the end of your thighs—and then set it down once the set is over. The biggest benefit of seated calf machines is ease of use. Because most of these machines work the same, the only difference here in ease of use is whether the machine uses dual loading pins on each side or one central vertical loading pin in the center. A single loading pin makes for faster and easier loading, especially in cramped quarters.

Comfort

Eventually, you may tire of that towel or bar pad digging into your thighs. Seated calf machines offer two comfort features—the seat and the thigh pads. Check the thigh pads under substantial load to ensure that it really is a comfort improvement over that towel or bar pad—otherwise, you are just paying for ease of use.

Capacity

Training alone, you can only load so much on a bar or hoist the heaviest dumbbell you have on your thighs, before capacity becomes an issue. Calf machines are designed to overcome this problem. However, many low end seated calf raise machines cannot handle much more weight than your loaded bar or heavy dumbbell, so make sure the machine's stated capacity can handle loads far in excess of whatever you can currently use.

Budget Seated Calf Raise ($0)

Go old school and use a barbell or dumbbell resting on your thighs, using the floor or a plate under your toes to increase the range of motion. If using a barbell, wrap a towel around the middle to increase the comfort of the weight sitting on your thighs.

Economy Seated Calf Raise ($50)

Upgrade to private school and use a barbell or dumbbell resting on your thighs, in conjunction with a calf block. If using a barbell, place a barbell pad (see, this is useful—just not for squats) around the middle of the bar to increase the comfort of the weight sitting on your thighs.

Luxury Seated Calf Raise ($150-$500)

Purchase a dedicated plate-loaded seated calf raise machine. Many Internet retailers sell these—just read the review comments and note the capacity and stability. You may need Olympic plate conversion sleeves as well. Oh, and you don't need a $1000 unit here—they offer no additional value over units at half the price, except perhaps baked enamel coated finishing.

Standing Calf Raise

Success tends to leave clues. Look at any professional dancer or Olympic fencing champion and notice the calves. Pretty impressive. Athletes like these don't typically perform any calf raises on dedicated equipment. What they do is essentially perform continuous repetitions of toe raises as part of their inherent sport each day for high volume.

Because you can easily accomplish standing calf raises using a calf block or plate lying on the ground, in conjunction with a dumbbell or power rack/barbell for resistance, the only need for a dedicated machine here is for quick drop sets—and I don't think that use warrants spending $300+ on a dedicated machine or consuming the floor space required.

What you do want to spend your time or money on here is the calf block. I'll talk about calf blocks in detail in the section on accessory equipment. However, for now, there are three things to consider for an effective standing calf raise:

Range of Motion

Perhaps nowhere else is range of motion so critical to provoking an adaptive response than with calf work. Walking only moves the calf muscles through half their range of motion. Therefore, we need to start our calf raises with our toes elevated above our heels—a 3" to 4" inch elevation works best for most, so look for that in a calf block or machine. Placing an Olympic plate on the ground and using that to elevate the toes will only give you about an inch or so of elevation, so the calf block or platform will definitely produce a more adaptive response.

Ease of Use

Look for calf machines that are easy to load and unload.

Comfort

This deals with two things—for machines, the pads that rest on your shoulders and for both, the shape and construction of the calf platform (or block). Ideally, your toes should rest on a calf platform that is slightly rounded and heavily padded with thick rubber. This allows you to perform calf raises in bare feet, or at least without shoes.

Budget Standing Calf Raise ($0-$5)
Grab a dumbbell for resistance and stand with your toes on a plate lying on the floor to increase your range of motion. Many a calf was built using standing dumbbell calf raises this way. Don't underestimate the effectiveness of this setup.

Economy Standing Calf Raise ($50)
Because you've already got a power rack and barbell (don't you?), add a calf block to engineer yourself a good standing calf raise setup.

Luxury Standing Calf Raise ($100)
The only improvement here is a rounded calf block that allows you greater range and the ability to perform these barefoot—which often produces a nice anabolic shock to the calves.

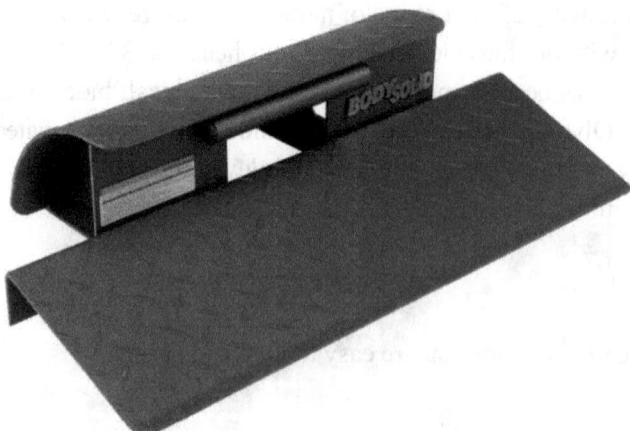

Leg Press/Hack Squat

Because squats (of all types) should comprise the core and majority of any successful leg training routine, then why do we need or want a leg press or hack squat machine, especially in a home gym environment?

Two reasons—for detrained individuals (and all beginners are detrained) or for times when the lower back involvement needs to be minimized (injury rehab, periodization, and mental breaks). I've found success (and a happy low back and fresh mind) when I perform a non-squat leg session about every four weeks. That's where I find my vertical leg press calling and the gains still coming.

A leg press or hack squat is still a superfluous piece of leg equipment. It's not necessary, but is a nice addition for both physical and mental respites, if you have the space and budget.

There are several types of leg press/hack squat machine to consider.

Leg Presses—If You've Got to Have One, Which is Best?

Like Border Collies, leg press machines come in all variety, but with a singular purpose—horizontal, angled and vertical, plate-loaded and weight-stack based. Which is best? Considering gravity, it seems logical that the vertical leg press is the winner here. It's also the type of leg press machine that most closely simulates a squat movement, with minimal involvement of the lower back. For many, this is a godsend. I can personally attest to this. I've used every type of leg pressing apparatus invented, from the original Nautilus leg press/extension beast (loved it!), to various horizontal weight-stack machines and most commonly, the angled plate-loaded variety.

For least low back involvement, the horizontal machine wins, but also requires an integrated weight-stack and a large amount of floor space—which home gym trainers typically don't have. Home versions of angled, plate-loaded leg press machines are available, but typically offer limited loading capabilities to the advanced trainer.

For the home gym bodybuilder, your best bet is a plate-loaded vertical leg press. The amount of resistance you'll use is typically just above what your working squat weight will be.

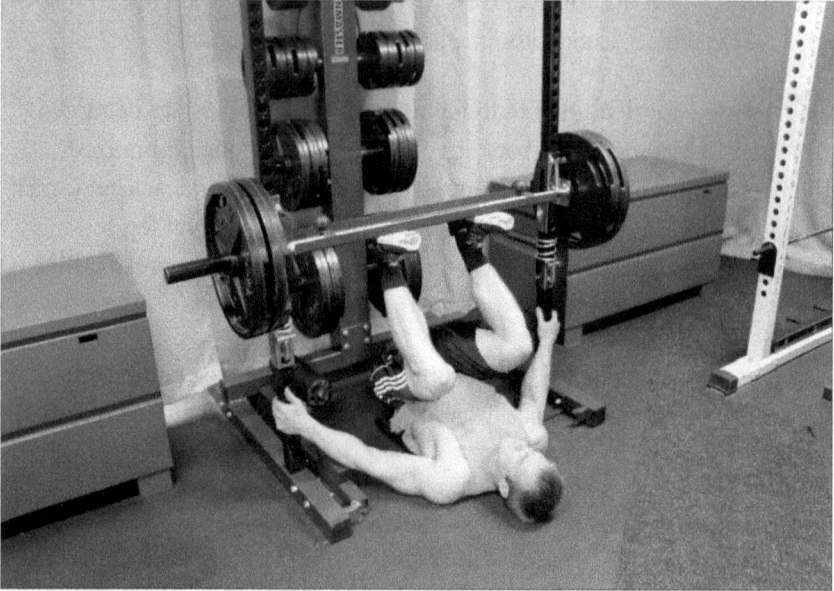

Combo Leg Press/Hack Squat Machines

Hack squat movements shift most of the involvement squarely on the quadriceps, with minimal to no activation of the hamstrings or glutes. This sled-based movement is popular in most commercial gyms because most people don't like to squat down to parallel or below with heavy loads on their back. But, because you aren't most people, you don't really need this movement at all.

However, if you are going to obtain a leg press machine, especially of the angled, plate-loaded variety, then you may want to consider a combination machine that converts between leg press and hack squat. This will save you space, give you two machine-based leg movements and still offer occasional relief to the low back. Again, these type of home-based units typically offer limited loading capabilities to the advanced trainer.

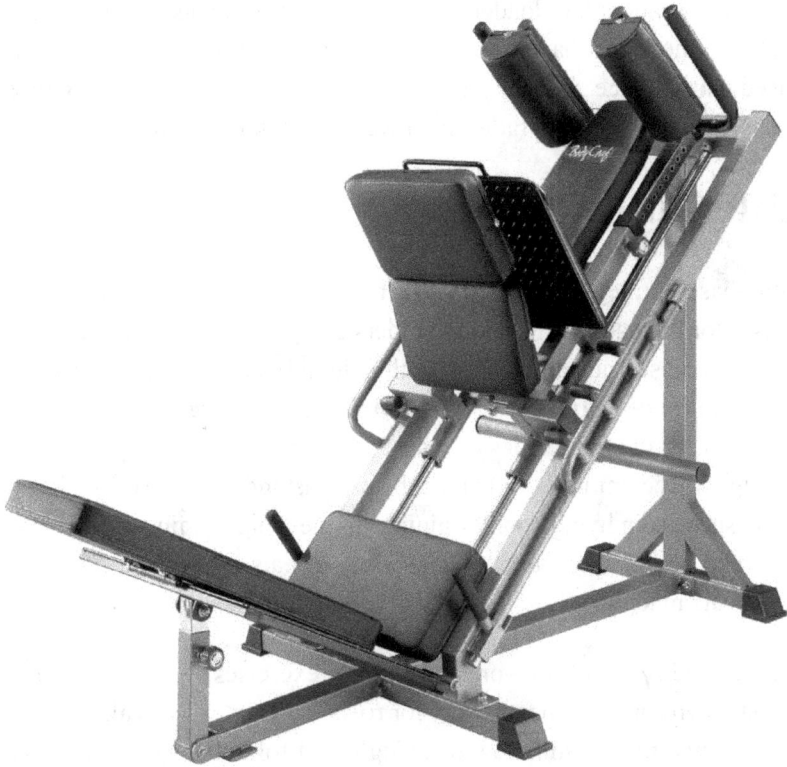

Remember, you can always perform the hack squat movement with the barbell held behind your back, old school, like Grimek, Pearl and Reeves used to do. Nobody laughed at their legs.

Budget Leg Press ($250-$500)
A plate-loaded vertical leg press is the most effective, space-efficient and budget friendly option for those looking for a leg press machine.

Economy Leg Press ($500-$1500)
Look for a used or low-end , plate-loaded combo leg press/hack squat machine from online boards or Internet retailers. These will take up about double the space of the vertical leg press.

Luxury Leg Press ($1500+)

Commercial-grade, plate-loaded leg press and hack squats machines are available to those that have lots of space of lots of cash. Your best bet is the used marketplace. Opt for plate-loaded versions of an angled leg press and a hack squat machine, rather than weight-stack based machines.

Cable Pulley System

A cable-based pulley system allows us to perform a large variety of exercises for the back, arms and shoulders using constant resistance. In fact, any exercise you can perform with a dumbbell, you can also perform with a cable (once again, Pearl's *Keys to the Inner Universe* shows us the way). Weaving the two modes of resistance into your training program—free weights (accommodating) and cables (constant)—is one of the keys to ultimate success in hypertrophy training. In the weight training game of rock, paper, and scissors, free weights always beats cables, and cables always beats machines.

Here, we need two pulleys—one set high for exercises such as pull-downs and pushdowns and another set low for rows, curls, etc. Typically, both the high and low pulleys combine into a single unit for home gym use.

Additionally, cable systems are available in two setups (standalone or as a rack attachment) with two loading schemes (plate-based and weight-stack based). Which you ultimately choose will have significant effects on the types of training and stimulus you can achieve.

Weight-Stack (Selectorized) Cable Systems

This is the preferred setup. Why? Because weight stacks allow you to rapidly change the weight simply by removing and inserting the selector pin. That allows you to incorporate advanced training techniques, such as drop-sets into your program. However, as they say, there is no free lunch. Weight-stack systems are far more expensive than their plate-based counterparts are. Additionally, most of these home-based weigh- stack units top out at 200lbs, which may be fine for most women, children and untrained men. More advanced trainers will ultimately require something in excess of 200lbs, especially for back exercises such as lat pull-downs and seated cable rows. Keep this in mind when deciding which to obtain.

Plate-Based Cable Systems

Although weight-stack cable systems are the holy grail of cable equipment, for home use and home budgets, plate-based cable systems are more practical, if less convenient and amenable to change the resistance quickly. What you'll want to take note of here is the total weight capacity that can be loaded onto the carriage unit. Again, look for units that can exceed 200lbs, with 250lbs and even 300lbs preferable.

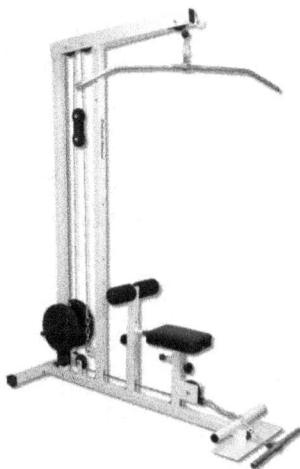

Many of these plate-based systems accept both standard and Olympic size plates, so make sure you get the Olympic size plate adaptors for the carriage loading pins. This is also where your micro-loading plates will allow you to progress in small increments—something that most commercial gyms do not offer with their cable apparatus.

Standalone Cable Systems

Standalone, weight-stack cable machines are the gold standard, and commercial norm, for incorporating cable training into your routine. However, for home gym trainers, they are relatively expensive (even with the plate-loaded variety), but much more importantly, they take up considerable floor space, especially if you are looking at dedicated units for a high and low cable setup. The dedicated plate-loaded cable machines also require room on each side of the unit for you to maneuver when loading plates. For our purposes, the much-more budget and space friendly alternative is the power rack cable attachment.

Power Rack Cable Attachments

Most power rack lat pull-down attachments are plate-loaded. This will be fine for most, but just remember to check the carriage's weight capacity and the presence of both a high and low pulley. Also, remember that some advanced training techniques, which require rapid resistance changes, won't be available to you in this setup. For those who can afford it, I recommend spending a little more for a weight-stack based pull-down attachment.

This is one of the areas that I guarantee you'll be glad you spent more in order to avoid the drudgery of loading and unloading plates, when you can just stick a pin in the stack. It's the accumulation of small conveniences like this that keep you relishing your home gym setup over the long haul.

Budget Cable System ($200-$400)
Get yourself a plate-loaded power rack pull-down attachment. This will open the world of cable training to you.

Economy Cable System ($400-$800, based on stack capacity)
Move up to a weight-stack based power rack pull-down attachment. Convenience awaits.

Luxury Cable System ($1000+)
Buy a standalone lat pull-down machine, preferably one with a weight stack. Most of these will include both high and low cables. For the ultra-rich, like my friend spending his Dave Dollars™, get *separate* machines dedicated to lat pull-downs and low rows.

Preacher Curl

Besides the Arm Blaster device (I'll get to that below), adding a preacher curl attachment to your home gym will probably do more for your long-term biceps development than anything else. Why? Because it forces you to isolate the biceps and minimize your ego (women don't seem to have this problem).

The preacher curl bench was invented by Harvey and Dale Easton of Easton's Gym in Hollywood. Legendary trainer Vince Gironda ("The Iron Guru") trained at Easton's while in his early, formative twenties. In 1948, when Vince opened his gym in North Hollywood he copied the bench and used it to great effect on one of his star pupils, Larry Scott. Scott's arms popularized the bench for all time.

You have two alternatives here—a standalone preacher curl bench (expensive in terms of budget and space) or the more popular preacher curl attachment for your adjustable bench. Based on similar effect, you can guess which one I recommend.

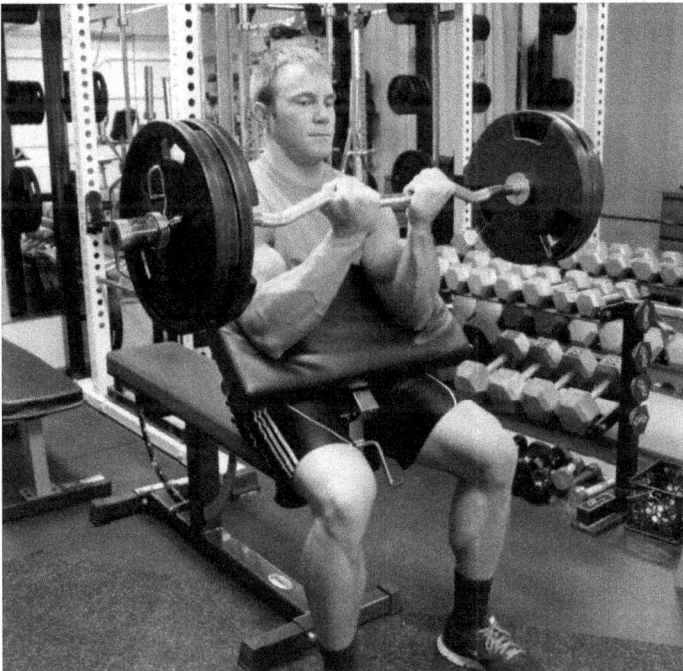

Budget Preacher Curl ($30)

Just use an Arm Blaster. Much cheaper with similar purpose and results.

Economy Preacher Curl ($50-$100)

A preacher curl attachment for your adjustable bench. Common, inexpensive and effective. Watch out for how the bench behaves when you are curling loads of weight.

Luxury Preacher Curl ($150+)

A standalone preacher curl bench. Better yet, if you're gonna go this route, do it right and get an honest to god Scott Curl bench. Beware and avoid the standalone plate-loaded preacher curl setups, otherwise you've just locked yourself into both a movement pattern and a specific application of that pattern. The preacher bench allows us to use bars, dumbbells and cables in a preacher curl environment. That's what we want.

Machines You Don't Need

Commercial gyms love machines. It's easy to see why. First, all those machines tell the novice, "hey, look at all we offer". This siren song has been playing since Arthur Jones first invented Nautilus. Ignore it. There are two central problems with most exercise machines.

First, they are designed for an "average" human—whatever that is. Typically, the manufacturer designs their machine line to conform best to a person about 5'6" to 5'8" in height. If you don't fit that profile, then the fixed movement path of the machine may not fit you correctly, even with adjustable seats.

Second, machines offer a single movement path or pattern, which may or may not adhere to your natural movement abilities. Body weight exercises, free weights and cables allow your body to move in its natural patterns.

Let's look at some of the most popular—and advertised—exercise machines and apparatus available that you don't need.

Ab Machines

This is probably my biggest pet peeve. Larry Scott noted that if you want to injure your back, an ab machine is probably the quickest and best way to do it. Other than an inexpensive ab pad (for increased range of motion), an ab roller, and perhaps some Hang-Ups, there isn't any so-called ab machine that you need.

Low Back Extension Machines

You see these all the time in commercial gyms. I'm not talking about hyperextension benches (which are fine), but rather those weight-stack based machines that provide resistance as you lean backward. Properly performed deadlifts, squats and good mornings will provide all the resistance, strength and hypertrophy that your lower back needs. Because you already have a rack, bar and plates, you have all the low back equipment you'll ever need.

Curl Machines

Most of these are preacher curl-based. If you follow the advice in this book, you have a preacher curl attachment for your adjustable bench—so you actually have something better, something that allows you to alter the mode of resistance (barbell, dumbbell, cable) as well as curling variation (supinated, hammer, reverse, Zottman). No set of curling machines can duplicate that.

Adductor/Abductor Machines

These machines are popular with women, but can be effective for men as well. However, there is absolutely nothing that these machines offer above and beyond what results you can get with squats and lunges. In fact, if you have a lat pull-down attachment for your power rack that has a low cable (most do), then you can purchase an inexpensive ankle strap (or make one yourself) for about $15 that allows you to duplicate the resistance movement of these machines.

Neck Machines

Yes, neck machines are nice—but do you really want to spend hundreds of dollars on a machine that just works your neck? Even if you are a wrestler, boxer, or football player?

If direct neck work is important to you or your sport, save yourself about half a home gym's worth of money and buy a neck harness that allows plates to be attached. Believe me, it's just as effective, if not more so.

Cardio Equipment

How important is cardio work to a bodybuilder?

Here's what noted strength coach "Maximum" Bob Whelan says about this in *Super Natural Strength*:

"Once you get over thirty, there is no excuse for not doing regular cardiovascular training…Your goal is not to 'look big' in your coffin."

Remember our discussion of health versus fitness? Well, cardio work is essential for good health. It's good for your heart, lungs and other essential body functions. For fitness, and bodybuilding in particular, it depends. If you are currently sitting at a relatively high body fat composition (and that could be as low as 12% for male bodybuilders and 20% for females) then cardio ratchets up the priority list, along with getting your diet under stricter control.

The problem with cardio training is how people approach it and the results it subsequently produces—typically from irrelevant to inappropriate and counterproductive, at least for our purposes. What we want to do is teach the nervous system the right lessons, with short periods of intense cardio, allowing the continuing promotion of muscular gains, while remembering our oath to health. We also have to remember the rule of metabolic specificity (you are what you do—are you a runner or a lifter?) and balance the role of aerobics in bodybuilding training—not an easy task, but necessary.

With that background, the inclusion of cardio equipment is an essential element to any serious healthy bodybuilding effort. Because extensive aerobic training has a negative effect on muscle size, strength and power, so we want to keep our cardio equipment's time investment, cost and space requirements to a minimum, recognizing that our time, energy and adaptive capacity are finite.

There are two problems with most cardio equipment—space issues and fit.

First, other than bikes, most other cardio equipment, such as treadmills, ellipticals, steppers, and rowers, take up a lot of valuable space in the home gym.

Second, the "right" cardio equipment is different for everyone. Most people get the best results doing what they enjoy. If that elliptical or stepper doesn't "fit" or accommodate you—if it doesn't move in a pattern that works for your body—then it's not going to work for you, becoming relegated to the clothes hanger life it wasn't meant to do. Obtaining cardio equipment that doesn't fit your body correctly will produce injuries, not results.

There's a third issue with cardio equipment, albeit one that can easily be overcome. This stuff can be expensive—at least the really well built, well-engineered models that adjust to your fit and can sustain an extended workload over many years. Although treadmills and ellipticals start around $400, the ones that work well over time usually include another digit in the price. This is the area where you really do get what you pay for. So, caveat emptor—if you opt for a bargain-bin treadmill, don't be surprised when it starts giving you trouble. Soon. When in doubt, type the make and model number of the cardio equipment you are pondering into a search engine, followed by the word 'review'. Then, read the reviews.

Because science now tells us that short and intense aerobic workout sessions burn fat better than long, slow steady state, it doesn't make much sense to dedicate a large portion of space or money to this activity, does it?

Let's see how we can mitigate these issues of space and accommodation and get a consistent, effective cardio workout that produces greater health and leaner bodies.

You & Nature

One of the best forms of cardio training is the one most accessible and obvious—outdoor movement, such as walking, hiking, jogging or running.

Marty Gallagher, strength coach extraordinaire, has been preaching and demonstrating this "phenomenon" of outdoor cardio for decades, through fast trail walking and the intermittent use of the Heavy Hands technique. Concurrently, former Mr. America Clarence Bass (author of the *Ripped* series of books) has clearly shown what daily walking can do to acquire and maintain a lean physique at any age.

If you are budget constrained, this is the form of cardio training that is always free.

However, outdoor cardio workouts aren't always possible, depending on your location, climate and changing weather conditions. Therefore, you'll need to equip your home gym with something for indoor cardio training for these situations.

Jump Ropes

Rope jumping is great whole-body cardio and a monster method for elevating the heart rate. The key is to perform this basic cardio training for extended periods of time—not just eight or nine swings of the rope until it snags your foot. Additionally, the rope does not discriminate—both low-intensity steady state and high-intensity interval training are there for the rope master to initiate. Adding in various jump patterns such as forward, backward and lateral movements also engages stabilizer muscles.

So, if jumping rope is so effective in conditioning, why don't we see more people at gyms—and more people in general—jumping? Because society tells us it's a kids thing and it's damn hard to perform for extended periods because it works so well. Remember, we're looking for safe, efficient and effective. That's a jump rope personified, so practice, practice and then practice some more.

Although jump ropes with weighted handles are nice, ones with weighted handles AND ropes are even better, because it provides a more dynamic effect as well as rotating smoothly around your body. That's important for both intensity and duration.

Weighted jump ropes are typically available in one-pound increments from 1-5lbs. This allows you to add some progressive resistance and progression to this simple cardio option.

The big downer here is that, for indoor use, it requires enough vertical space for rope clearance—something you may not have in a room, shed or basement. Therefore, this may not be a year-round option for you, but that's ok—remember, we want to change our method of cardio from time to time (4-6 weeks) just as we change our weight training—unless exercise longevity is not important to you. For the limited budget group, maybe let the time and weather dictate the mode—rope jumping in nice daytime weather, kettlebells at night during the snow, rain and cold.

For apartment dwellers, unless you land with light feet or live on the ground floor, your neighbors below you may not appreciate this form of cardio.

One final concern—it's an impact-based activity and some may not tolerate this well, especially for extended periods. Even more reason to use periodization in all aspects of training.

Budget Jump Rope ($0)
Surely, you have a length of rope lying around somewhere. Cut it to an appropriate length and go.

Economy Jump Rope ($10-$20)
A simple commercial-grade rope with handles.

Luxury Jump Rope ($20+)
Get yourself a couple commercial ropes—some weighted at various levels with ball-bearing handles. One with a nice built-in counter offers the instant ability to track progress here with both time and reps. Couple this with a heart rate monitor and you've got yourself a human performance lab for conditioning.

Now, let's move on to the more popular cardio choices. Because many people spend a lot of money on cardio machines every year and then never use them, you can find a plethora of great deals here.

Kettlebells

Yes, kettlebells are for cardio too. The benefits here include non-impact movement, no need for extended ceiling heights, and minimal space and time when compared to other forms of cardio training. In addition, it's just damn cool to learn, execute and master conditioning movements with tools that have been used for centuries.

We're talking relatively lighter kettlebells here, performed for continuous repetitive movement, typically with one arm for five minutes, then the other for the remaining five. No breaks, no putting the bell down. This is the Russian *girevoy* style training that will transform your body. As a bonus, because lighter kettlebells are lighter on your wallet, you can obtain world-class cardio equipment inexpensively—equipment that will outlast you and not break down. This is where Pavel would say, you have no excuse comrade!

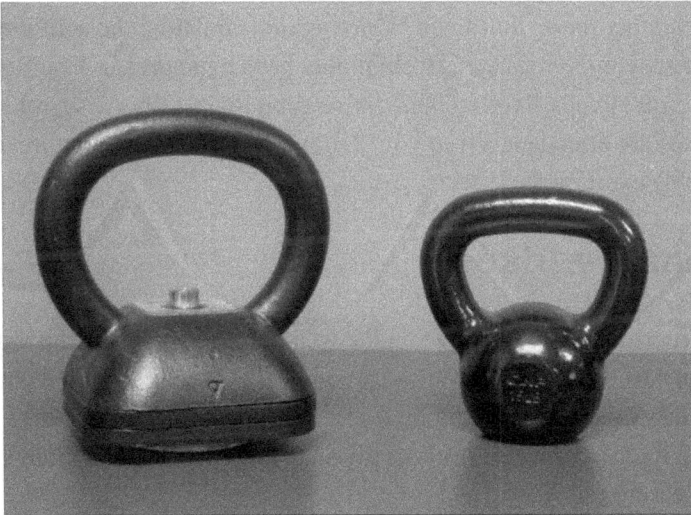

Although an introduction to kettlebell training is beyond the scope of this book, I can point you to the Internet, and specifically YouTube, for lots of free, quality kettlebell instruction.

Bikes & Stationary Bikes

Bikes and stationary bikes have long been the fat-burning, cardiovascular equipment of choice for bodybuilders, starting in the 1950s. Biking provides a zero-impact heart elevating activity that is nice to your knees and joints. It also gives your upper body a break, something that may be welcomed by those recovering from injury, those recovering from a heavy squat or deadlift session, or those with lower back and knee issues. However, because there is no free lunch, removal of the upper body from stationary biking also decreases the adaptive stimulus, given a set time period. However, there are alternatives that add this back in.

Let's take a look at your biking options and the advantages and disadvantages of each.

Bicycles

You remember these, don't you? Once again, emulating the activities and movements you performed as a child may have even greater benefits as an adult. If you already have a bike, you're good to go. Otherwise, reliable used bikes are abundant, given your fellow man's seeming abhorrence to sustainable exercise.

Stationary Bikes

These are a great alternative when the weather turns brutal or the traffic seems unsurmountable. They also take up little space in a home gym, which makes them ideal given their effectiveness, especially in their adaptive ability to provide both steady state and high-intensity interval training cardio (HIIT).

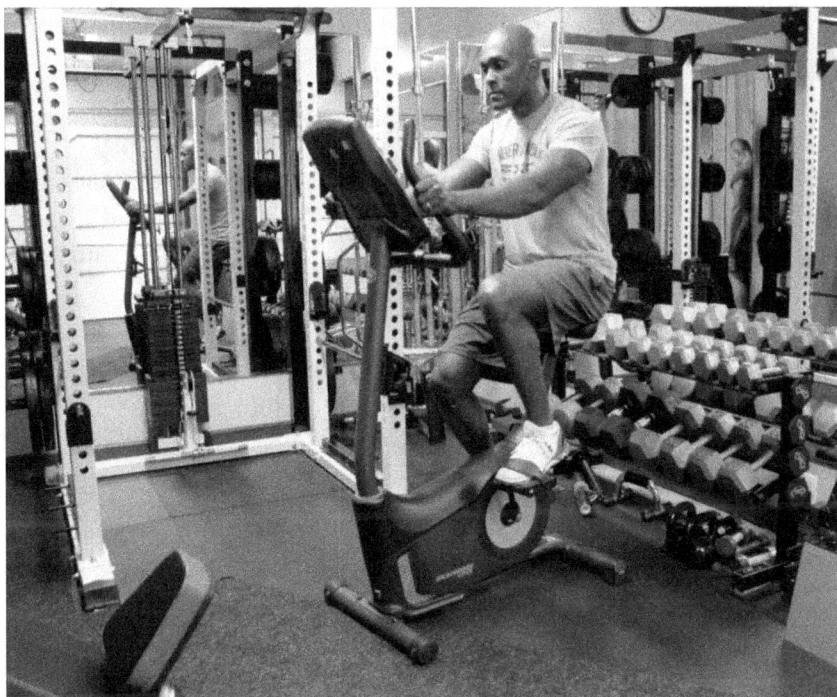

In the past, you had little option here—an upright exercise bike with a hand-cranked resistance wheel bearing down on the single bike tire. Now, the options are many.

Types of Resistance

You can still obtain old-school hand-cranked resistance exercise bikes—they are cheap and effective— however, monitoring, and recording your progress often becomes an exercise in subjectivity, especially when multiple users are involved. When you remount the bike for another session, perhaps after your wife worked out, how do you set the resistance to the exact same level (or slightly higher) using an analog-based resistance knob? In short, you can't. That's the basic problem with serious use of this type of resistance bike. However, manual resistance bikes tend to last forever.

In order to provide a more entertaining and accurate resistance challenge, modern stationary bikes combine digital settings coupled to an electronically triggered magnetic flywheel for exacting and variable resistance. These bikes provide the same basic cardiovascular effectiveness as the old manually controlled resistance bikes, but allow you to more accurately set and record your resistance level per session. This makes a big difference over the long haul in producing a more effective cardio-based adaptation for your body and your health. The downside here? The weak link is the electronics. If the electronics fail, the bike essentially becomes near useless, with no method to control the resistance.

Finally, air-based resistance bikes, such as the famous AirDyne models, offer another alternative. As expected, they use air for resistance—the faster you pedal the greater the resistance. A side bonus, especially in hot, humid environments is that your pedaling produces a human-powered air conditioner. For cold climates, you may not be so enamored. Although newer units do provide simple electronics that measure time, distance and estimated calories burned, they are still an analog-based resistance device. Your effect provides the resistance level, not a computer. As to longevity, air-bikes typically enjoy the same longevity as their old, manual resistance cousins, although the used prices here are higher because these bikes are not as common.

Upright Bikes

Once you understand the types of resistance offered by various stationary bike designs, you have another basic consideration—do you want to pedal the bike in the traditional upright position, or in a recumbent position?

Upright bikes are what you grew up with. They feel 'natural'. They also support manual, electronic and air resistance modes, take up less room than recumbent bikes and are less expensive. So why consider a recumbent bike?

Recumbent Bikes

These bikes place you in a laid-back reclining position, which offers ergonomic benefits.

Due to the reclined position of your body, comfort and activation of your glutes is increased, and stress on the lower back and arms decreases. However, the disadvantages of this design, compared to upright bikes, include constant positioning (you can't stand up to 'sprint'), less athletic skill transfer to road bikes, increased expense and floor space requirements.

They also don't offer the next option we'll look at.

Combo Bikes – Upper & Lower Body

Some upright bikes offer upper body inclusion via synchronized arm levers, used in conjunction with the foot pedals. Recumbent bikes do not offer this level of full body involvement. Because cardio becomes more effective as you engage more areas of your body, these upper/lower body combo bikes make excellent choices for the home gym bodybuilder. Think of them as bike-based elliptical machines, but ones that take up far less space and consume less dollars from your wallet.

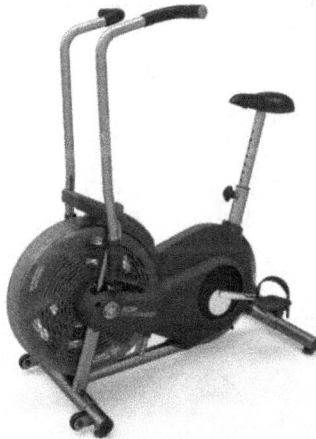

What about dedicated upper body bikes?

These hand or arms-only bikes are not good for general cardio use. Why? Because our goal in any type of cardiovascular exercise is to involve as much of the total body as possible. This is why cross-country skiing remains the absolute king of cardiovascular exercise. Arm bikes involve only the upper body and relegate the lower body to spectator status. They are useful for those who have lower body impairments and want to elicit a cardiovascular effect, which make almost all other types of cardio inaccessible.

Using Your Road Bike Indoors

There is one alternative for indoor cardio that uses your existing road bike and has direct skill transfer to that mode—the use of an indoor bike roller trainer, such as a full, two-wheel frame or the more compact, affordable and safer one-wheel stands.

This may be an attractive option for those looking to provide multiple cardio units simultaneously, with minor expense and room space (when not in use—hang those bikes on the wall!), using your own bikes.

Regardless of which type of bike you choose (if you choose a bike at all), they need to be adjusted to fit each individual person properly (you can't adjust treadmills—therefore, purchase carefully there).

For upright bikes, watch for bike seats that are too far back—causing you to lean forward into the handlebars. Leaning forward on cardio equipment provides some rest for your body. Some studies have shown that this forward lean and support of the upper body can reduce the effectiveness of your cardio sessions by up to 20%. Just like there is no crying in baseball, there is no resting in cardio—at least if you are really playing baseball or are serious about your cardio.

Budget Bikes ($0-$50)

If you can't find a good, used road and/or stationary bike at a yard sale or on the Internet, then you aren't looking hard enough. They are everywhere. You can probably get one of each for $50, although you may need to clean them up and perform some minor repair.

Economy Bikes ($100-$400)

Affordable, quality upright stationary bikes are available used and new on the Internet, especially at major retailers. Read the reviews before buying, or better yet, try them at a store, then buy where the deal for the bike you like is best. This is where I landed for my primary piece of cardio in my garage gym.

Luxury Bikes ($400+)

Consider an air-powered or recumbent bike (if you have the floor space). A Schwinn AirDyne is one of the gold standards across the decades in human-powered cardio performance, adaptation and results.

Treadmills

I'm not a big fan of treadmills for home gym cardio work. Why? Two reasons. There's this thing called 'outside' that has an unlimited treadmill (with unlimited variety!) and in times of excessive heat, cold, rain, or snow, it's a good idea to perform a different type of cardio activity— periodization is not just for weights—this cardio periodization will have your body thanking you over the long haul.

However, if you insist…

Treadmills do have several things going for them—accessibility and convenience.

I've already mentioned that vigorous walking can dramatically alter your body fat composition, given a proper diet is in place. Gallagher and Bass showed us this. Treadmills are the most accessible method for walking when the outdoor variety is out the door. Similarly, amping the intensity with jogging and running in the dead of winter or during a driving rainstorm becomes possible.

Another form of accessibility and convenience is sometimes not as evident—you can put the treadmill in the same room as a TV and combine the love of television viewing with some old-fashioned movement. So, while *The Walking Dead* is on, you can walk right along with the zombies—or, better yet, try to stay ahead of them. Thirty or sixty minutes will pass quickly. This setup also encourages additional cardiovascular training frequency, which your heart will thank you for, and allows us to remove the cardio equipment from the home gym and regain that space for more progressive resistance activity. (As a general rule, three days per week of cardio activity is the bare minimum for health, 5-6 times per week says you're serious about fat loss, and seven-day per week cardio aficionados don't completely understand the concepts and process of recovery.)

When looking to purchase a treadmill, pay attention to these important details—deck length, incline ability, motor capability, and space requirements.

Deck Length

The deck (running surface or walking belt) should measure about 80 inches in length and 20-22 inches in width. Sizes smaller than this may impede or alter your natural walking or running gait, especially as your height exceeds the norm. You already know if that represents you or not. Cheaper treadmills often scale the deck length down—that's one of the reasons they cost less.

Incline Ability

Walking, jogging or running on a flat surface represents the lowest form of terrain intensity. Performing these same activities on inclined surfaces increases the intensity. Check to see if the treadmill has the ability to incline, and if so, how many degrees of incline are possible. The more, the better.

Motor Capability

In electric treadmills, the motor is everything. The amount of horsepower the motor can generate ultimately determines the maximum speed and incline possible.

Right off the bat, one problem with most non-commercial treadmills is their inability to achieve speeds near your full exertion—speeds that are necessary for high-intensity interval training (HIIT). Look for the continuous horsepower number—you need a treadmill with a minimum of 2.0 continuous horsepower to meet your increasing conditioning needs. Also, and I hate to say it, but it is a truth, the heavier you are, the more motor horsepower you'll need to power the deck. So consider that, if you need to.

Space Requirements

Because most treadmills are roughly three feet wide and six to eight feet long, they occupy a lot of space. For practical home use, look for models that fold up when not in use, reducing the amount of square feet required from about twenty to three.

What About Manual Treadmills?

With manual treadmills, you power the belt, not a motor. Typically, a weighted flywheel provides relatively smooth movement. This drastically reduces the price. However, these units are limited in practice to individuals that weigh less than 250lbs, have no lower back issues and want to walk, not jog or run (manual treadmills often exacerbate low back pain). If you fit these requirements and goals, this may be a viable and inexpensive option for you.

Availability

Electric treadmills are common in the used market, because most people purchase them new, and then discard them months later when well-intentioned exercise plans fade and the units remain, taking up space.

Here's what you need to do when evaluating a treadmill—used or new:

- If the unit folds up, make sure it folds up and stays folded up.

- Get on the unit, set it to a slow speed and try walking, then jogging, then running. Make sure you can stride normally and there is enough width to the belt that you don't feel you will fall off.

- Crank up the speed to the maximum for a couple seconds and see how the motor performs.

- If the unit offers incline ability, test it through all the incline settings. Then, test it again with the motor at full speed.

- Check all the electronics. With computer-controlled cardio equipment, the electronics are the Achilles heel.

If the treadmill passes all the tests, make sure the price is competitive relative to its condition and capabilities. The Internet will help you here.

Ellipticals

Other than cross-country ski machines (remember Nordic Track?—they are awesomely effective), elliptical machines are the godsend for individuals who prefer or require a non-impact cardio activity that incorporates the full body.

As with bikes and treadmills, there are some unique characteristics to consider here—stride length, footplates, resistance levels, capacity limitations and space requirements.

Stride Length

The stride length is the most critical feature here. Look for machines with adjustable stride lengths that reach at least 20". Anything shorter and you may find yourself moving with short, quick, choppy strokes. This is not good for your body. This is also where most inexpensive units reside—in the land of 16-18" strides. If the stride length is not listed, be wary—and always take a tape measure to verify.

Foot Plates

What can be so concerning about the platform your foot goes on? Take a couple steps and notice your ankle. It does not remain in a fixed angular position as you walk. Elliptical machines that have fixed foot plates while the armature rotates creates an unnatural walking or striding motion. Look for articulating foot plates—those that allow your ankle to move freely as you stride forward. When we are simulating a natural movement, we need the machine to play along with us.

Resistance Levels

In short, you want more than one. Because we are progressing in all aspects of training, aerobic as well as anaerobic, you need the availability of some way to increase the resistance. Most elliptical machines will include upwards of 8-12 "levels". Look for those machines and avoid the manual resistance ones, which use your stride speed as the only variable.

Capacity

Most home-based ellipticals have a capacity of 250-300lbs. If you are near these numbers, make sure the unit can hold you and is stable when moving at full speed.

Space Requirements

Space requirements for elliptical machines can vary greatly, but because there are no folding units here the minimal amount of space you'll need is about twelve square feet (think 3' wide by at least 4' long). Heavier, more capable units can occupy at upwards of six feet in length. They are big machines, which is why I don't have one in my garage gym. If you can dedicate space in another room for it, then this consideration falls down the importance list.

Steppers

I know several competitive bodybuilders who use the StepMill™ for cardio and glute work during contest prep. However, you'll be hard pressed to duplicate the level of effectiveness of this commercial machine at home. Here's why.

Most home steppers use adjustable-resistance hydraulic cylinders to increase the level and intensity of effort. Commercial steppers use motors that drive step pedals or rotating staircase steps (the StepMill™). More expensive home units do have motors and step pedals, but the motors are significantly less powerful than commercial units. Besides the difference in function (rotating steps versus step pedals) and power (hydraulic cylinders or low-powered motors), home steppers typically do not allow for the same range of stepping heights as their commercial brethren. This is the real downfall. We've seen this with short deck treadmills and minimized stride length elliptical machines. Restricting your natural, full-range of motion will restrict your results and may alter your biomechanics in a negative way.

You should see a pattern emerging by now. Each variety of cardio equipment, while varied, has common concerns, along with a few unique considerations. Steppers are no different.

Step Height Range

If you have a chance, play the crazy guy or lady and take a retractable tape measure to the nearest commercial gym and measure the height between steps on the StepMill™ (if they have one) or the step pedal range for the other steppers. Note this, then when shopping for a home step machine, pull out your tape measure and compare. This will give you the clearest comparison of effectiveness between machines, followed by operational smoothness and resistance capabilities.

Resistance Levels

At first, especially if you haven't been performing step-based training, the use of a step machine will be effective even at low levels of resistance. This will quickly change. Make sure that even at the highest level of resistance the machine offers, that the resistance is at the "almost impossible" level. Because, one day this will be possible. At that point, duration becomes your sole traveling companion.

Capacity

Most home steppers can hold people up to 250lbs. In reality, some of the folding step machines become somewhat unstable beyond 200lbs.

Space Requirements

Some of these home step units fold up. That's a big plus. However, if they fold up, it most likely a hydraulic cylinder unit, with lower weight capacity and step range. Keep that in mind as you weigh the tradeoffs.

Availability

Due to the popularity of home-based treadmills and bikes, used step machines are not as common. If you do find one, it's bound to be a hydraulic cylinder-based unit. Likewise, these days sporting goods stores are stuffed full of elliptical machines and treadmills, with a few upright and recumbent bikes peppered in. Comparing step machines becomes a little more challenging.

Rowers

Rowing machines provide effective low-impact cardio work that involves most of the body. They are equally suited to both steady state and interval-based training. Additionally, rowers can strip body fat and improve your heart's performance and your level of cardiovascular conditioning beyond your wildest imagination.

However, here—unlike with the bikes, treadmills, ellipticals, and steppers—there is a clear, singular choice for durability and performance—

the Concept 2 rower. Sure, this might set you back a grand (new), but you'll be hard pressed to find another indoor cardio machine that will provide these results for decades without breaking down. Every collegiate and professional sports training facility worth their salt has at least one of these—probably more. Olympians have trained on them for decades and you may have seen them on ESPN at the World Crossfit Games.

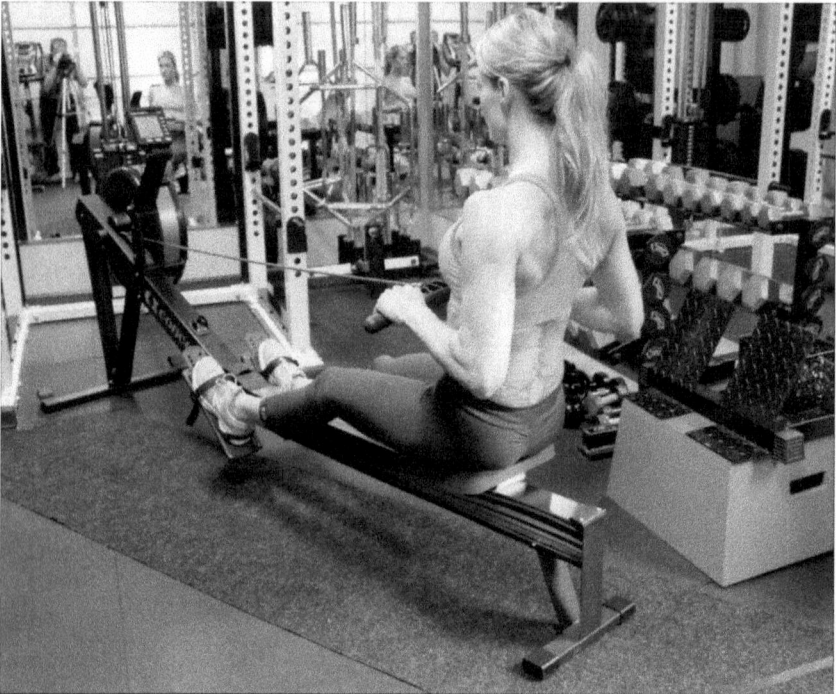

Another huge benefit here—although Concept 2 rowers have been around for decades, even the earliest models are upgradable to the newest technology. Yearly maintenance is as simple as oiling the chain. They are built like tanks, designed for hard and consistent punishment, yet if something were to break, parts are available for all models. This is the one true rower, the one that rules them all. I think you can tell I like it—and yes, I have one.

Space Requirements

In use, the Concept 2 takes up an area of two feet wide by eight feet in length. However, when not in use, it folds in in half vertically to occupy a small 2x3 foot space. That's six square feet for one of the finest pieces of cardio equipment on the planet.

Availability

As mentioned, you can buy a new Concept 2 for a thousand dollars or seek out a used unit. However, be aware that used prices here run about 20% less than new. Supply and demand rules. These are serious machines, such that supply is relatively low, and demand is high by those in the know. If you find one that is anywhere near half off the new price, don't hesitate. It will probably be gone within hours.

Hybrid Devices

In your quest to obtain a piece of cardio equipment, you will probably run across hybrid devices, such as bikes that also double as ellipticals, or ellipticals that can be set to step mode. Here's my advice—avoid these. In practice, they resemble Crossfit—marginal to good in each activity, but not excellent in both. You are much better off buying a machine that dedicated to a single type of task.

• • • •

Summing up all your cardio options, here are some overall recommendations for your home-gym conditioning arsenal.

Budget Cardio ($0-$50)
Get outside and walk, jog, run, bike, skate—whatever. If that's not possible, a jump rope or a couple kettlebells will fit the bill for not many bills.

Economy Cardio ($50-$100)
You should be able to find a used stationary bike online or at a yard sale. Use any leftover cardio funds to get some kettlebells and a jump rope. You

now have at least four options for cardio—outside training with your feet, indoor biking, jump rope and kettlebells. All for under a hundred bucks.

Luxury Cardio ($400+)

At the low end of luxury are some nice stationary bikes and some decent used treadmills. For those with serious desires and serious money, you can't beat a Concept 2 rower.

Training Journal

Originally, I was going to list a training journal under the Accessory Equipment section, but a journal isn't an accessory, it's essential—just as important in many ways as the dumbbells, bars, plates, bench and rack. The training journal is the most important tool in the bodybuilder's toolbox. If you don't have a training journal then you aren't training—you're just working out. There's a big difference. In my small part of the world, I've got some training partners, like Dave, Andrew and Jake—none of whom keeps a training journal—instead, relying on me to reconstruct memories of past workouts they completed. Of course, this is horrific, even with my good long-term memory, because my journals reflect my performances—not theirs. In essence, they are relying on my expertise and judgment to carve out their path to success. What happens when I'm not there?

The real key to sustainable use of a gym—particularly a home gym—is to see your progress manifest itself in hard numbers. As the amount of weight you can lift improves on particular movements, your physique will improve and your enthusiasm remains sustained.

Now, here's the really important part for long-term success (in anything). Take some time each year to review your journals. Therein lies the gold. Dan John talks about mining his journals like a prospector seeking clues to unusual performances. Do the same. Don't repeat past failures. Sure, John McCallum delivered to us the *Keys to Progress*, but reviewing your training journals are the real key to your individualized progress. Failure to do this is tantamount to following in the footsteps of Sisyphus, as you make the same mistakes repeatedly. Remember and reinforce the successful insights in order to form a long-term lesson plan for your body.

So many smart coaches and trainers have written, discussed and even shouted about the importance of the training journal, so my voice here would seem to be lost in a crowd of advocates. However, it's been my experience that no one is listening, or is even in the room. Please don't make that mistake.

Budget Training Journal ($1)

It's called a spiral notebook. Add a pen and you're all done. It's useful if it has as many pages as days of the year you'll train. Aim for 250-300 pages and you won't run out.

Economy Training Journal ($10-$20)

Okay, you can buy a journal that's specific to weight training. The only reason to do this is to save some input time and provide consistency across workout recordings.

Luxury Training Journal ($20+)

Is there a luxury training journal? I'm not sure I've ever seen one. In any case, I can't imagine they would add that much additional value for recording training sessions and performing training analysis—unless it's with an electronic journal.

Accessory Equipment

The basic equipment for bodybuilding—dumbbells, bars, plates, an adjustable bench, rack and cable system will cover about 90% of everything you need. To get at the remaining 10%, there are several pieces of accessory equipment you may want to add gradually to your gym. The key words here are 'accessory' and 'gradually'.

In this section, I'll discuss these accessories—you can decide which, if any, you ultimately want to obtain.

Shoes

A lot of us work out in running shoes or some other fashionable sports-based footwear. That's not an ideal thing, at least from an optimum weight training perspective, and here's why.

Think about the shoes that you currently wear when training. Are they optimized for propelling weight upward (standing presses, deadlifts, squats, upright rows, etc.)? Chances are you are wearing shoes with compressible heals, something that doesn't provide a stable platform, and that absorbs the initial force you intended entirely for the weights.

Note that I am not suggesting the use of dedicated weightlifting shoes, such as those specifically for squatting, deadlifting or Olympic lifting. For bodybuilding, you really don't need those, and in fact, they become a hindrance because you need to remove them for exercises that require extreme ankle flexion, such as calf raises. In fact, lifting exclusively in weightlifting shoes for the variety of bodybuilding movements may alter your biomechanics in an undesirable way. Think of bent-over dumbbell laterals with raised heel squat shoes. Not optimal.

What's the ideal shoe? How about none. God gave you the best lifting platform—your bare feet. This is another benefit of the home gym. Although the local gym owner will surely run you out if you lift barefoot, the freedom of your home gym opens this option. Your foot has the surest angle of attack and most stable surface for lifting heavy loads. If you insist on covering this greatest asset, consider something that minimally impacts this natural gift—hard, flat shoes, deadlift slippers, the thinnest, barest of flip-flops or even those newer five-toed 'barefoot' running shoes. In addition, heed the cautionary advice—but not the 'solution' of the naysayer—and be careful when picking things up and putting them down near your feet regardless of what you wear. Not many shoes can protect your foot from a falling 100lb dumbbell or 45lb plate.

I use either bare feet, water shoes or a general-purpose sneaker with a wide, flat and solid heel for almost all of my weight training and cardio, depending on what I'm doing and what I feel like. For squatting, I do use a dedicated squat shoe, but that's because my leg training involves prodigious amounts of squatting of all types, and they were a birthday gift from my wife and they work great—for the intended purpose.

Budget Shoes ($0)
Lift in your socks or bare feet. Good enough for Arnold, good enough for you. Watch how you lower or drop plates and dumbbells. Safety first—if you tend to drop things, wear shoes or find a different activity.

Economy Shoes ($20+)
Chuck Taylors, military boots or anything with a hard, non-compressible sole that provides a platform for progress.

Luxury Shoes ($100+)
General purpose cross-training shoes with good stability, and a solid base. Get some dedicated weight training shoes and squat shoes. You won't regret it.

Chalk

Good old magnesium carbonate. It's helped everyone from Mary Lou Retton to Arnold Schwarzenegger, as well as the guy in the gym last week get that fifth rep on the deadlift.

Chalk is a safety device. It helps absorb sweat and provides you with a non-slipping, secure grip when holding bars and dumbbells, especially in humid home gym environments. Chalk also decrease callus formation by filling your skin folds. Personally, I find calluses beneficial to lifting so that may be something you mediate. You can buy a decade's worth of gymnastics chalk on the Internet for about $15, so go do that.

The big gripe about chalk in commercial gyms, and why it's so often banned, is because it tends to get everywhere. Because this gym is your gym you will have to dictate how much of a concern that is for you (if it is, then there are chalk balls you can purchase that leave only minor residue). I suggest using a bucket or large plastic container to serve as your chalk urn. More upscale lifters may want a commercial chalk stand.

DIY Chalk Buckets

There are a plethora of options for making your own chalk receptacle, from empty protein powder containers, plastic buckets, coolers, Tupperware, and zip-lock bags, all the way to plastic potting planters coupled with pipe and plywood or dirt tampers as a weighted base. These options will set you back from zero to about thirty bucks.

I leveraged the plastic popcorn bucket that was formerly full of caramel during my vacation into my chalk bucket. My daughter Julia even spray painted the bucket to match the color scheme in my home gym and wrote 'CHALK' on the lid with magic marker. That's one way to erase the guilty memories of binging at the beach along with getting the family involved in ownership of the home gym. Bonus—because she has actively engaged in gymnastics for years, she knows what to do with the chalk!

Weightlifting Belt

The purpose of a weightlifting belt is to stabilize the spine by adding additional intra-abdominal pressure to your abs—thus, an appropriate belt, worn correctly, is like extra abs. (In fact, your ab's job is to do the belt's job of containing and maximizing intra-abdominal pressure so you can remain rigid while lifting heavy weights.)

When it comes to belts, most lifters will head to the nearest Walmart or sporting goods store, grab a belt that fits properly around their waist, and proceed to the checkout. However, there are a few things to think about here in order to make an intelligent decision.

Leather or Nylon

Leather belts provide a stiffer, less forgiving support than their nylon counterparts. The choice here really comes down to personal preference, although the leather belt has endured legions of pounding over the past century and remains a true companion.

Locking Mechanism

Weightlifting belts are secured around the waist by either a prong, quick-release mechanism, a lever or velcro. Most belts use the prong design (like any typical pants belt) and allow you to get the belt as tight as necessary. However, in some cases your waist and the belt may not be in agreement—if there isn't a hole right where you need insert the prongs, then the belt will either be too tight or too loose. Because you don't want to continually play the part of Goldilocks when lifting, make sure to try on this type of belt before purchase to ensure the exact fit you need. If your waist increases or decreases, this can disrupt things (and may be another indicator of health or fitness). Single-prong belts are easier to adjust but have only a single point of failure. Double-pronged belts are more common and have built-in redundancy. Keep that in mind. I've used the same leather double-pronged belt for the past fifteen years with no problem. It's been a reliable companion when I need it.

A quick-release belt obviates this issue by providing a truly custom fit by allowing you to adjust the belt to the appropriate diameter and lock it in place (typically with a lever). Both of these types of locking mechanism are secure.

Lever belts are common in the powerlifting world and provide absolute tightness and security. However, they require disassembly of the locking mechanism if you need to adjust the size of the belt.

Velcro is use as the locking mechanism for nylon belts. I bet you're already asking yourself, "how secure is that". Most are surprisingly secure, although I've witnessed many an occasion when I was spotting a heavy squat and heard that familiar sound of the Velcro loosening or about to release. I'll stick with my prong-based leather belt, thank you. At least you can check the integrity of the locking mechanism before use. Velcro belts are ultimately limited in their force exertion capacity versus their leather-skinned rivals.

Thickness

Most leather belts come in two diameters—10mm and 13mm. Powerlifters typically use the more rigid 13mm belts. Because we are bodybuilders, the more common 10mm is fine.

Width

Finally, we come to width. Weightlifting belts are available in widths ranging from two to six inches. Bodybuilding belts are wider in the back and narrower in the front. I recommend a belt with a four inch width at the back—this will provide the most versatility for both heavy squats and deadlifts.

So, the big question is—when should you wear a belt?

The easy answer is—if you need it.

Consistent use of a weightlifting belt, without proper ab training, will create a weak link in the midsection. So, just say no to the lifting belt, unless you are performing some seriously heavy overhead pressing, squatting or deadlifting. Even then, you may not need it.

You can also use the belt itself as exercise apparatus. For example, if you have a low cable mechanism, take your weightlifting belt and buckle it. Now, attach the buckle to the low pulley. Lie down on your back in front of the pulley and hook your feet in the belt. Pull your knees toward your chest to work your abdominals and hip flexors in progressive fashion. Just be careful not to allow your feet to slip out of the belt.

One caution here—don't use a weightlifting belt as a dipping belt. It will break. Trust me.

Budget Weightlifting Belt ($20)

Any standard issue leather weightlifting belt from Walmart, the Internet or a sporting goods store will work fine. Get one with a four inch width at the back and not the wider six inch models. Novice lifters can get by with a nylon belt, but you won't be a novice for long and the leather belt will carry you on throughout your training career.

Economy Weightlifting Belt ($40-$80)

Move up to a more rigid, thicker belt from a quality manufacturer, such as Schiek or Rogue. These will have heavy-duty prongs and construction and can handle the heaviest loads that a bodybuilder will use.

Luxury Weightlifting Belt ($100-$150)

The only move up here from a good economy belt to luxury is to get one with a custom design or your name embedded into the back of the belt. If you go this route, you had better be able to walk the walk, because your belt will be doing the talking.

Dip Belt

Once you get proficient at performing multiple sets of 15+ reps of dips or pull-ups using your body weight, it's time to make those dips progressively harder. You'll need a good dip belt for this. Don't try to use your weightlifting belt with a rope or chain. As I mentioned previously, it will break.

Dip belts are even simpler devices than weightlifting belts. It's just a belt with some type of chain or nylon that hangs down in front to attach weight to. What is important here are capacity and fit.

All god dip belts will state their load capacity. If it doesn't, assume it can hold about 100 pounds. High-end dip belts can hold upwards of 3000lbs (I'm not kidding), although I haven't met the man (or woman!) who can handle that or even attempt it (don't!).

As to fit, I'm talking to the men here. Because dip belt chains (or nylon) can hang precariously close to the family jewels, it's important to look for a dip belt that provides a wider, and more forgiving, space between the chain, the dangling weights and your manhood. These wide-set dip belts are available and I highly recommend them. Yes, I have witnessed some narrow escapes concerning dip belt chains and amateur circumcision.

Budget Dip Belt ($0-$10)
Make one yourself. There are many DIY dip belt plans on the Internet, most using chain, rubber tubing and carabineers. You probably have some of this stuff lying around. In addition, you can make it to fit.

Economy Dip Belt ($20-$40)
Sure, there are plans on the Internet for DIY dip belts—but why? That same Internet has some good dip belts for sale in the $20-$40 range.

Luxury Dip Belt ($50-$75)
What's the difference between an economy, run-of-the-mill dip belt and a luxury belt? Fit, capacity and durability. Economy belts will accommodate loads of up to 100lbs. They also stray particularly close to a man's most valuable possessions. High-end dip belts fit more appropriately, and offer load capacities that exceed anything you've ever imagined, short of a World's Strongest Man Competition. They will last forever.

Lifting Straps

Weightlifting straps replace your inherent grasping strength. As such, the use of straps can hinder or propel your bodybuilding results, based on your strategic use of them.

Mark Rippetoe provides a succinct explanation of the correct use:

"Straps are a good example of equipment you need for some things but shouldn't use for others. Straps are good for heavy shrugs, the kind performed in the rack with a hundred pounds more than your max deadlift; exceptionally heavy shrugs are not possible without straps. They are good for deadlift assistance stuff, like rack pulls from below the knees to lockout that can be done with weights too heavy to hold for a set of five."

When searching for a pair of lifting straps to add to your home gym toolkit, the concerns here are durability, length and securing method.

Durability

Cheap, run-of-the-mill straps will eventually break. I've seen it dozens of times. Because most lifting straps are canvas, the durable ones are made from heavy, thicker canvas. I suggest spending more and buying the heavy-duty, thick canvas powerlifting straps. They will last your entire lifting career and you can check this item off your forever list.

Strap Length

Lifting straps are available in lengths ranging from 12" to 18". What's important here is your hand size, strap length, and the ability for you to consistently wrap the strap around the bar or dumbbell in order to achieve a secure grip. So, get the correct length for your anatomy.

Securing the Straps

There are two points of contact for securing straps—around your wrist and around the handle of the weight. With traditional powerlifting straps (essentially two pieces of cloth), you slip your wrist through the loop in the strap and simply wrap the remaining length of canvas around the bar or dumbbell. Although this works well for powerlifters who perform relatively low rep schemes, for bodybuilders who perform a variety of rep ranges—some relatively high (think 20 rep sets)—it's useful to use straps that contain a few enhancements.

By enhancements, I'm talking about lifting straps with Velcro closures around the wrist and with dowels at the end. The combination of steel buckle and Velcro keeps the straps secure around the wrist, whereas the dowel ensures the ability to lock the strap in place with relative ease. Once locked, the strap remains tight for the duration of the set. Releasing a dowel-based strap is equally quick and easy.

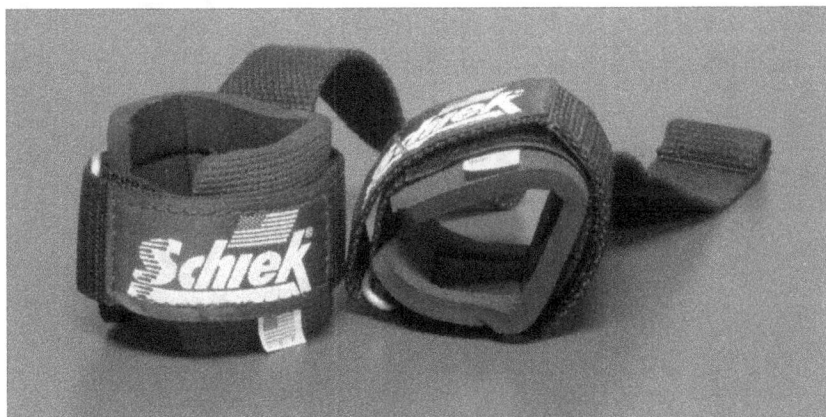

Budget Weightlifting Straps ($10)

A set of traditional canvas-based straps are cheap, relatively reliable over the short-term, and are available just about everywhere. Just remember, you will have to replace these eventually as they start to wear, then tear.

Economy Weightlifting Straps ($20-$30)

Instead of a cheap pair of straps, invest more upfront and get a heavy-duty set of canvas straps with Velcro closures and a dowel at the end. If you don't like the Velcro or dowel, there are many heavy duty straps available with just the Velcro or without any of that fancy stuff.

Luxury Weightlifting Straps ($25-$40)

Really, the luxury strap—one made of the most durable canvas from a top vendor, such as Inzer, is for the competitive powerlifter and not the bodybuilder. But if you must, they really aren't much more expensive than the economy models.

Thick Bars

Until recently, if you wanted to improve forearm, grip and overall strength with fat bars (barbells with large circumferences or dumbbells with thicker handles), well that was an expensive option. Now, with the availability of rubberized bar and dumbbell handle clamps, such as Fat Gripz™, this becomes an affordable and recommended piece of accessory equipment. For about $40, you can transform *all* of your bars, dumbbells, chin bar, and cable bar attachments into thick-based versions. I repeat—all of your stuff for about $40. That's home gym nirvana.

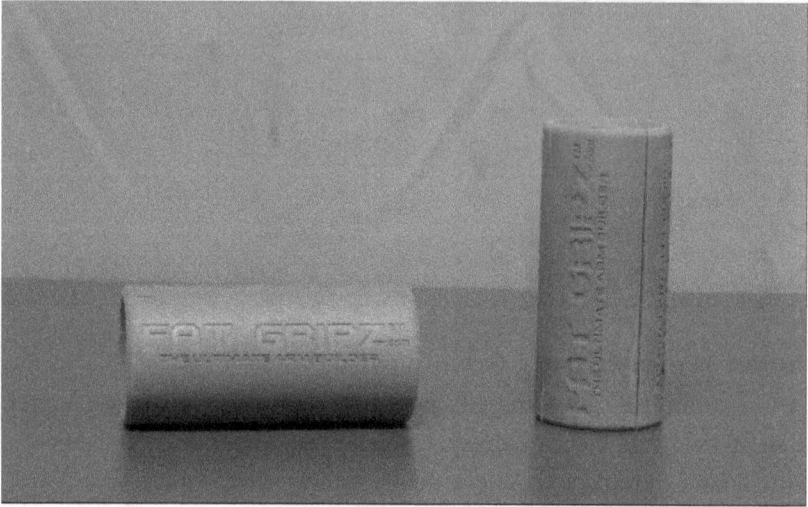

Just remember—don't use Fat Gripz™ and lifting straps at the same time. I've seen it, don't do it. Think about it—one negates the other.

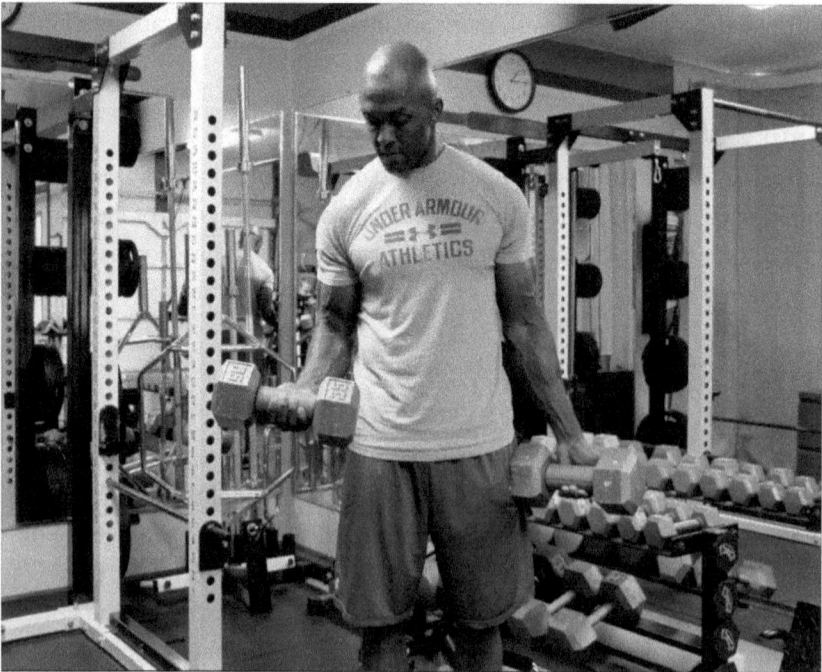

Budget Thick Bars ($40)

Rubberized bar and dumbbell handle clamps, a la Fat Gripz™.

Economy Thick Bars (various)

If you have access to old pipe, tractor axles, or similar thick handled apparatus, then you can use those in conjunction with lifting chains (I talk about those shortly) for progressive-resistance thick bar training.

Luxury Thick Bars ($300+)

Every type of barbell and dumbbell is available in various thick bar configurations. Things get expensive quickly here.

Ab Wheel

The ab wheel is one of the cheapest and most effective pieces of training equipment you can purchase. For about $10, you get a super-simple, effective means to strengthen the core and abs with a side treat for the lats. In fact, the ab wheel mimics the key ingredients to a proper pull-up: tight abs and an explosive movement near the finish. Along with the jump rope, this simple, inexpensive device clearly meets our objectives of safe, efficient and effective equipment. Great for those who have mastered the plank—it takes planking to the next level with a moving plank. Did I mention, it's super effective and super cheap?—around ten bucks. Get one.

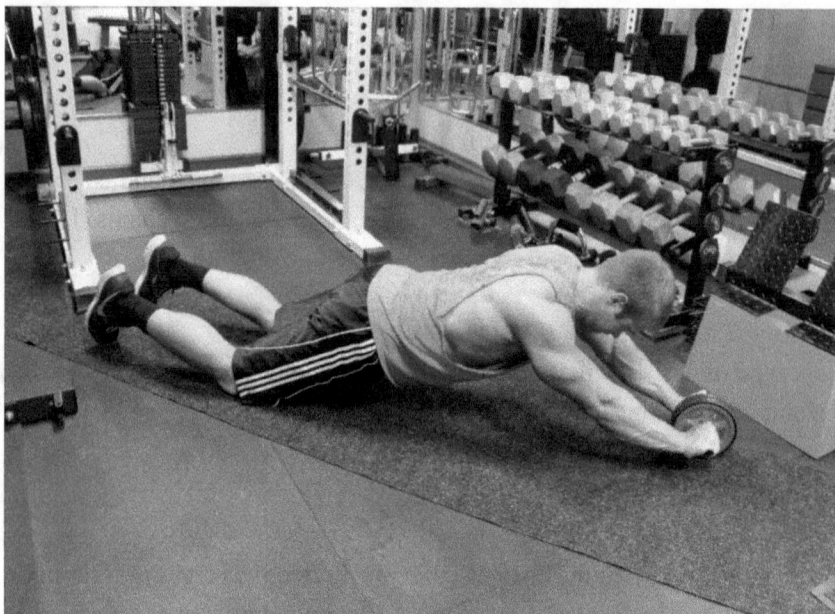

Budget Ab Wheel ($0)

You can use a barbell to perform your ab wheel rollouts. Try loading the bar with 10lb or 25lb plates for this. The 2.5lb and 5lb plates might not work, depending on the type of collars you are using. Spring collars will necessitate using the 10 and 25lb plates, because the smaller plates do not have enough diameter size to allow for a smooth bar roll with spring collars attached. For the masochists, try working up to the 45lb plates, or even multiples of 25s and 10s. Remember, even with ab rolling, we are still concerned with progressive resistance.

Economy Ab Wheel ($10)

At $10 new, this is probably the lowest cost piece of economy equipment you can buy.

Luxury Ab Wheel ($20-$30)

I guess you could spend upwards of $20-$30 for a fancier ab roller, one with a wider wheel or other high-tech options. However, does it work more effectively? I don't think so. Unless you are a really big guy that requires a steel version to avoid a face plant, stick with the budget or economy options here.

Calf Block

In order to achieve complete development of the calf muscles you need to move them through a full range of motion. Walking or running uses only half of the calf muscle's range. Therefore, for us home gym dwellers, you need a calf block to get at that other half.

Proper, baseline calf blocks should be 3" to 4" inches high, allowing a full, natural extension of the calf. They should also offer a non-slip surface for the toes and be capable of handling heavy loads far in excess of your body weight.

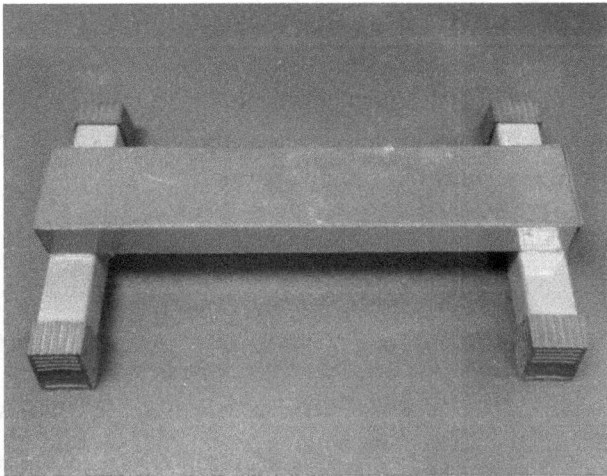

Higher quality calf blocks offer some minimal padding (typically rubberized), allowing for the use in socks or bare feet. Truly exceptional calf blocks have a slightly contoured top, rather than the standard flat surface, allowing for completely natural movement of the bare foot under load. This often leads to greater flexibility, stretch and thus calf growth.

Budget Calf Block ($10)
Try building one yourself. Construct a DIY calf block with some 2x4s or a single 4x4, wood screws and some non-slip adhesive. For those of you with about five minutes of spare time, just screw a larger piece of plywood (12"x18") onto the 4x4—and done. There are many good ideas for DIY

calf block construction on the Internet. Build this correctly and it's as good as the economy option.

Economy Calf Block ($40)

New, steel-based commercial calf blocks are heavy duty, plentiful and unsurprisingly similar to the DIY wood designs.

Luxury Calf Block ($100)

Only a few manufacturers make these heavy, high-end contoured steel calf blocks. Most double as squat accessories, but let's ignore that function. We want this for the contoured shape and the treasures it offers.

Cable Attachments

There are a plethora of attachments available for your high and low cable pulley system, a core group of which are useful, whereas others remain dubious. Here are the ones you should consider.

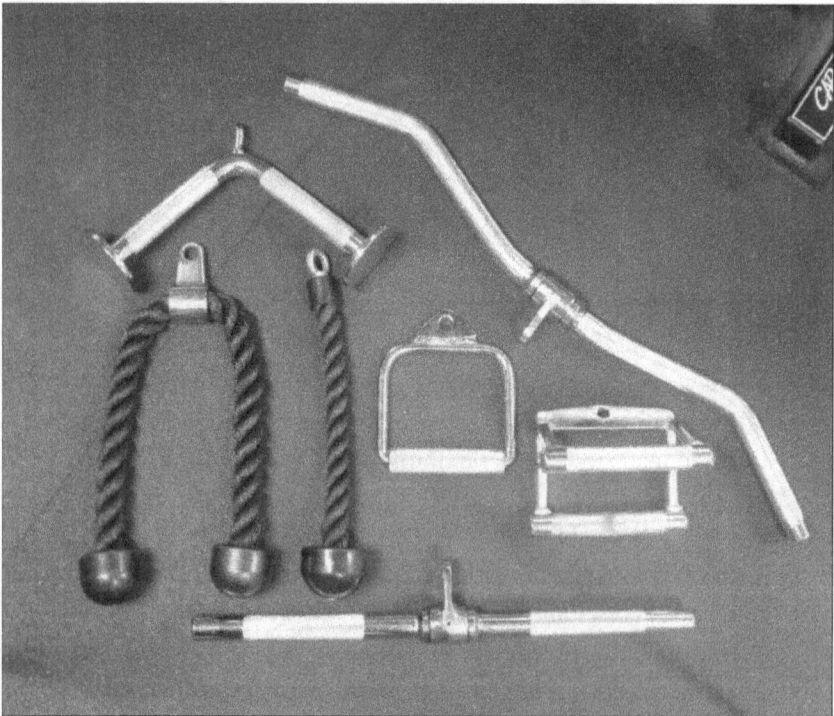

Lat Pulldown

The standard 48" lat pulldown bar is the cornerstone of cable attachments. This single addition will allow you to perform a plethora of cable-based exercises beyond the pulldowns, including tricep pushdowns, all kinds of curls, rows, upright rows, and front raises. It's the king of versatility for cable systems. This attachment should be in every cable owner's toolbox.

Things to be aware of here are length, knurling and shape.

If you have a particularly wide shoulder structure, you'll want an equally wide pulldown bar to match—otherwise, you might find your grip width limited by the bar's length.

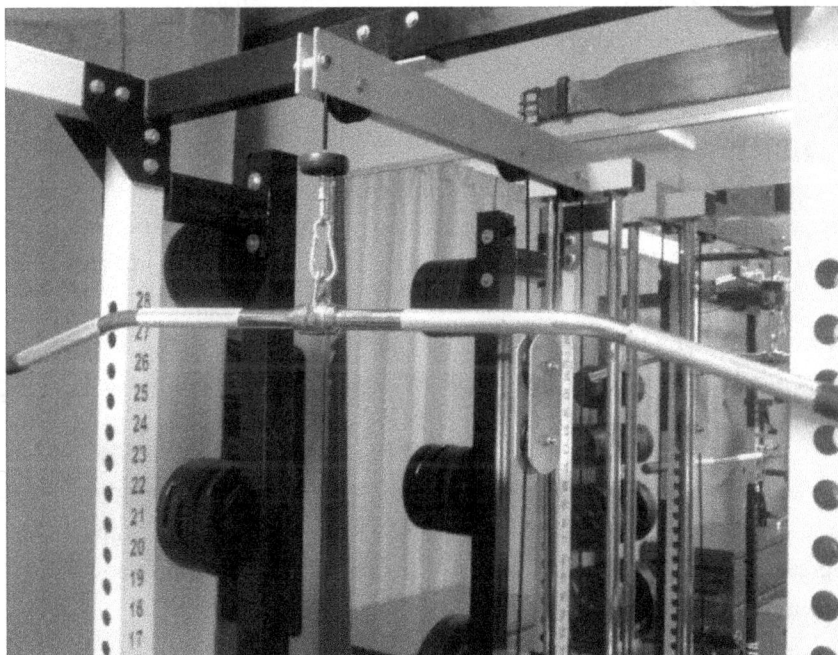

Most pulldown bars either have a rubberized coating along the bar or at the endpoints—we don't want this. Rubber will eventually tear and rip off, leaving a nice, shiny area with absolutely no grip whatsoever. Get a pulldown bar that has no rubberized coating anywhere (this rule applies to all cable attachments), with ample knurling along the bar, particularly at the endpoints and along the straight portion. Ideally, a pulldown bar with knurling along the entire length is the goal, providing grip anywhere you might want to place your hands. Because a pulldown bar offers a multitude of uses, length of knurl becomes important here. Additionally, try to match the depth of knurl to your preference. Because I like a deep, rough knurl, I bought attachments that offered this. I've found that used sporting goods stores are ideal for finding pulldown bars (and other useful types of attachments), as well as sampling the knurl.

Finally, pulldown bars come in various shapes, including completely straight (like a barbell), or with the common downward angle at each end for the traditional grip area. Again, if you have wide shoulders, make sure that the width of the bar is appropriate for you when gripping the downward angle area, and near the end of the straight bar. This will provide the greatest versatility with grips, something that becomes important for avoiding repetitive stress use, enhancing periodization, and providing longevity in lifting.

Upside Down Lat Pulldown

Larry Scott explained the importance of a pulldown bar with upward angled handles in his book, *Loaded Guns*. In brief, by positioning your hands in that upward angle, it forces the elbows outward and helps to spread the scapula and focus the stress on the lats. Try it now by holding your hands in that position and simulating the action of a pulldown movement. The difference in effect should be immediately obvious.

Don't try to rotate the bar of a standard lat pulldown attachment to this angle—with load, it will quickly rotate downward and possibly injure yourself. Dedicated upside down pulldown bars do not contain a rotational attachment element, and remain fixed in that unique position.

Because this type of specialized lat pulldown bar is differentiated only at the endpoints, the remainder of the bar is just as versatile as a standard lat pulldown bar. However, because these bars are much less common, their price is typically higher than the standard pulldown bar. If you do run across one in a used sporting goods store, buy it.

Triangle attachment

Small, triangular bars are useful for pushdown movements, especially for targeting stress to the lateral (outside) head of the triceps. Again, no rubber here and look for good knurling.

Short bar

There are a multitude of short cable bar options, including simple 20" straight bars, longer 30" bars, and various models with neutral-grip handles and even rotational (Supra) handles. Here, you can get as fancy as you want.

What you do want is to make sure the bar rotates—otherwise, things like curls get difficult, as the bar will want to rip out of your hands (or rip the skin on your hands) much like the old one-inch standard size barbell you fooled around with as a teenager.

I recommend getting two short bars, cousins to your Olympic barbell and EZ Curl bar setup. One straight and another EZ bar shaped will provide versatility, periodization, and wrist relief for most of your curling, pushdown and rowing needs.

Handle

A single, closed handle attachment is useful for performing unilateral pushdowns, curls and rows. Again, make sure the handle rotates and the knurling is appropriate.

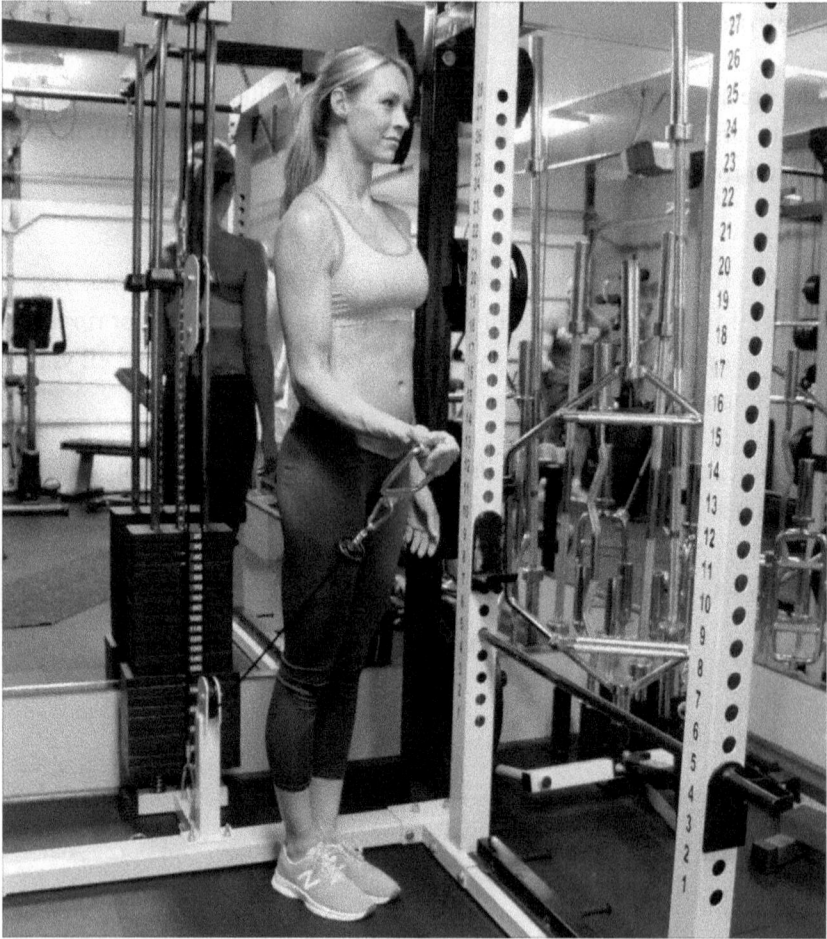

Ankle Strap

I don't use ankle strap attachments, but my wife does. If adduction, abduction, and leg kick movements are important to you, these are what you need (you can also sit on a bench and use them for leg extensions). Once attached to your ankle and the low cable, they do a good job of simulating those popular adductor and abductor machines at the gym. Be sure to get two of them so you won't have to continually remove and add the strap to each ankle as you train.

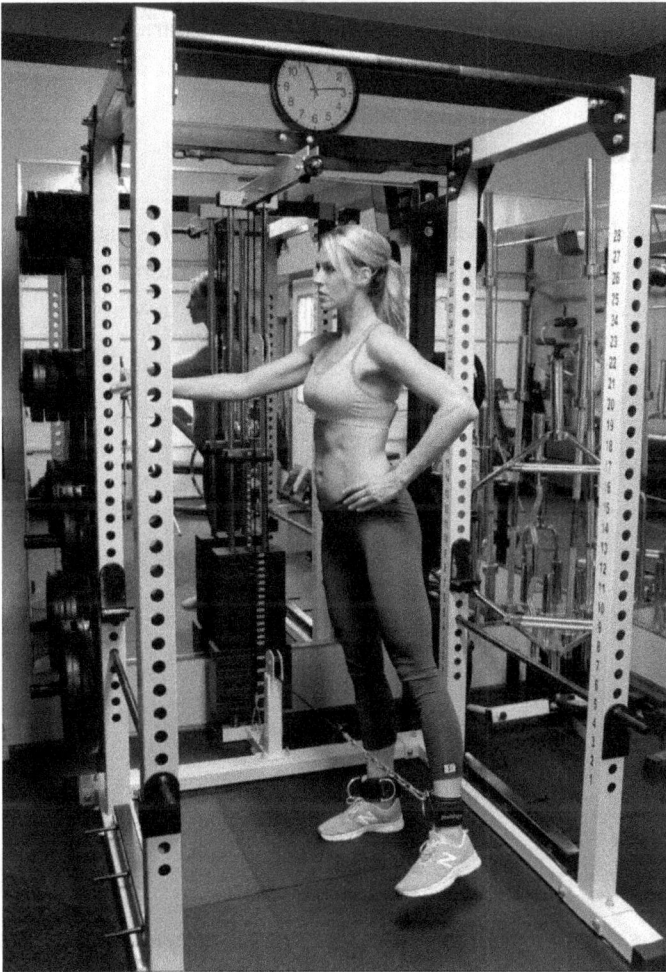

Budget Cable Attachments ($20-$50)

Start with the cornerstone of cable attachments—the versatile lat pulldown bar. Used ones are inexpensive, whereas new ones aren't much more, which allows you to shop around for that desired length, knurl, and shape.

Economy Cable Attachments ($50-$120)

Besides the lat bar, add a short EZ curl bar and a handle attachment. This will provide you with grip variety and unilateral versatility.

Luxury Cable Attachments ($150-$250)

Get 'em all. Lat bar, upside down lat bar, a couple various short bars, a handle and two ankle straps. Joe Gold would be proud.

Landmine

A landmine device, coupled with an Olympic barbell is useful for two things—pushing and pulling. You can perform unilateral pressing movements with this, as well as T-Bar or unilateral rowing.

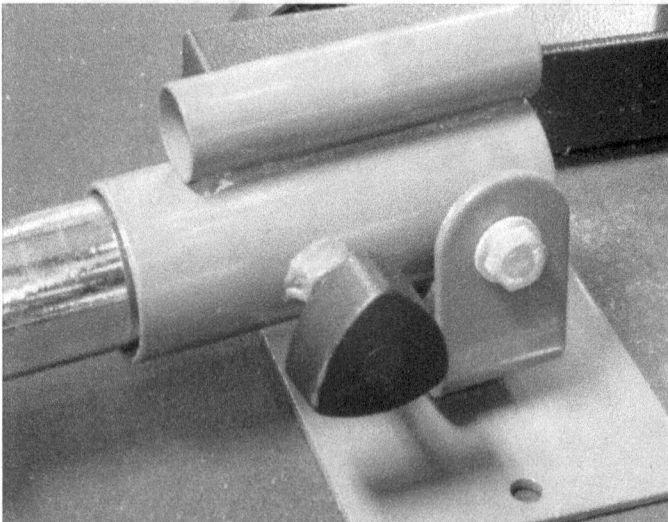

For it's versatile ability to transform barbell movements into unilateral exercises, I recommend adding it to your home gym.

Budget Landmine ($0)

OK, so the budget version doesn't even use a dedicated device. Just secure two 25lb plates on one end of the Olympic barbell and load up the other end with your working weight. The smaller plates at the far end of a seven-foot long Olympic bar, coupled with the laws of physics, will keep that end anchored to the floor (a folded towel under those weights also keeps it from rolling around). However, some lateral movement at the base may still occur, which is why I like the next option.

Economy Landmine ($40)

Buy an inexpensive landmine adaptor for your dumbbell rack or power rack. Make sure the adaptor fits the frame size of your rack. These are available from many retailers on the Internet—you're not going to find them in sporting goods stores.

Luxury Landmine ($150-$250)

A dedicated landmine unit with one or two bar attachments is commonplace in performance training centers and some commercial gyms. If you want to copy this, note that the heavy base ensures it won't move and the two-bar option is useful for alternating unilateral presses. All of this comes with a price.

Plyometric Boxes

For our purposes, we won't by using plyometric ("plyo") boxes in the traditional manner. Here, we want at least a paired set of them, for things like belt squats, box squats, high benches, forearms curls, rear delt laterals, and prone rows. Step-ups can be useful as well. In particular, the box squat, an often-overlooked exercise, allows for precisely measureable progress, providing an automatic depth indicator. This eliminates subjective squatting. The box also provides a bonus in confidence and security.

What you'll need is two plyo boxes of the same height. This is necessary for placing your flat bench on top of the boxes in order to construct a poor man's high bench. (Flat utility benches that are in excess of 30" in height are hard to find, and when you do find one, they are not surprisingly expensive. Additionally, in a home gym, they take up precious floor space.)

You can purchase pre-built metal or wood plyo boxes, wood box kits, or completely construct your own. DIY plans for these boxes abound on the Internet, and I've included one below. Regardless of your source, there are some requirements and guidelines to follow here.

First, the absolute requirements—the plyo box must be stable, flat and well built. It must be able to handle a load twice your body weight. Second, the recommended height should be 12"-14". This height accommodates flat utility benches at a height that permits unimpeded rows and laterals, and is a good base for box squats. Finally, ensure that the landing area will completely accommodate the feet of your bench, so measure those and note the specs for the box. My 12" height Rogue boxes have a 19"x19" landing area, which I verified beforehand was the exact width of the feet of my Adidas flat utility bench. For comparison, adjustable squat boxes typically have a 18"x18" landing area, so I'm pretty close there.

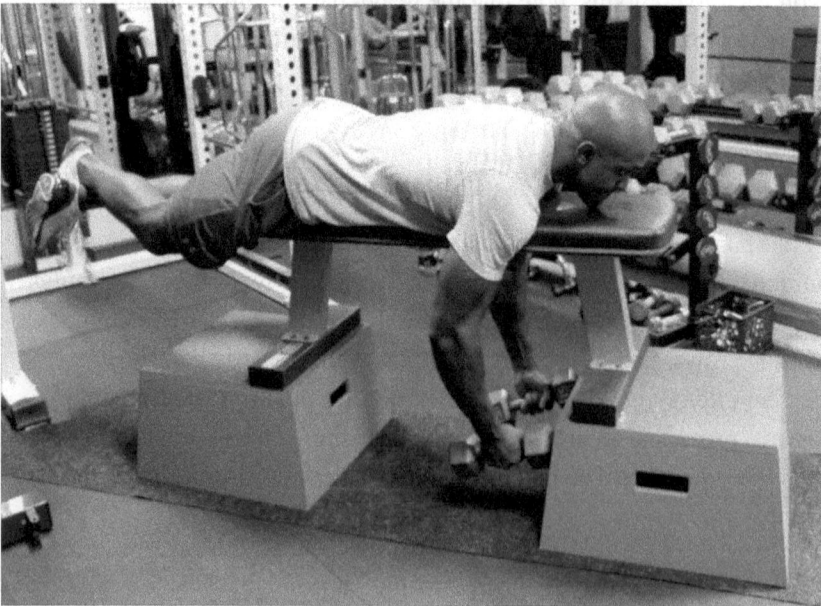

A final note about using a fixed height plyo box as an adjustable squat box: Employ the Louie Simmons' method of box squatting. Use extra three-quarter inch rubber mats (cut up an extra horse stall mat) under the box to adjust depth, as appropriate. This will allow you to modify the height of your box above and below its base height, essentially creating a low-cost adjustable box squat bench.

As promised, here's a typical plan to make your own plyometric box. Double the materials and duplicate the steps for a set.

DIY Plyometric Box

Cost: $20 per box

Materials:

(1) ¾" plywood sheet (4ft x 8ft)
(1) box of screws
(1) bottle of Gorilla Wood Glue

Step 1: Cutting
For a box of the recommended 12" height, you'll need to cut the following dimensions:

Top: Cut a 18.75"x18.75" square
Sides: Cut four side panels at 21.5" (base), tapering to 19" (topside) with sides at 11.25".

Step 2: Gluing and Screwing
Now that all your pieces are cut, you just need to glue them and screw them together. Anywhere wood touches wood, use glue. Start with the base and one side. After applying the glue to the connecting edges, place a screw about every 2-3 inches around the entire box. Overkill now helps ensure safety later.

Budget Plyo Boxes ($20 per box)
Make 'em yourself out of plywood, screws and wood glue.

Economy Plyo Boxes ($50-$75 per box)

Commercial wood plyo boxes that you screw and glue together. I got mine from Rogue.

Luxury Plyo Boxes ($125-$300 per box)

Get yourself a nice adjustable squat box. You'll need two to elevate a flat bench. Lucky bastard.

Chains

I know what you may be thinking—competitive Powerlifters use lifting chains in their training, not bodybuilders. Correct. But ignoring this valuable piece of equipment can limit the genetic hypertrophy potential of bodybuilders as well. We like people that train with open minds—that's usually what promotes progress.

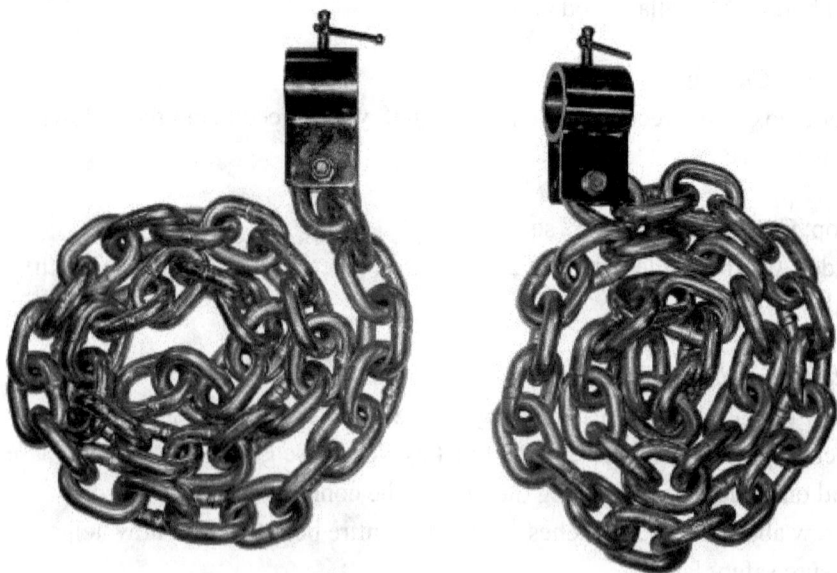

Lifting chains help develop strength and stability, which eventually translates into additional muscle gain. A myriad of exercises benefit from using chains—not just the typical squats, presses and deadlifts—but also isolation work with laterals and extensions as well. You'll probably think of more.

In most exercises, the movement becomes easier at the top where you are at your strongest. Unlike bands, which provide constant resistance, adding chains provides accommodating resistance to this natural strength curve. It helps push you past plateaus by allowing you to use more weight as the lift progresses and provide additional overload at the top of the movement. It also helps teach you to apply force throughout the entire movement and not decelerate near the end. I've also seen people use chains as quick accessory equipment for push-ups, chins and dips. Just drape them around your shoulders or torso and you're good to go.

Finally, chains can assist with injury rehab by taking pressure off those areas and providing reduced stress on joints, if used properly. For example, they can take pressure off the elbow joints at the bottom of extensions.

So, after you've bought into the effectiveness of chains for hypertrophy training, the logical question becomes—what weight of chain should you get? Typically, your current training loads answers the question. If you can lift about 200lbs, then a set of 20lb chains is reasonable. I like to use this 10% estimate when selecting chains and I think you'll find it effective as well.

Budget Lifting Chains ($0-$50)
DIY chains are the way to go here. A quick Internet search for 'DIY weightlifting chains' will turn up lots of good ideas. Most boil down to obtaining some used heavy-duty towing chains. Just throw the chain around the bar, secure with a carabiner, and you're all set. Check junk yards and auto repair centers as sources for inexpensive used chain. Also, most home improvement stores sell heavy chain by the foot.

Economy Lifting Chains ($100-$200)
Most large Internet retailers, such as Amazon, sell weightlifting chains in various weight increments with the big benefit of free shipping. These dedicated lifting chains include integrated collars, which simplifies the job of securing the chain to the bar.

Luxury Lifting Chains ($200+)
For bodybuilders, optimized zinc electroplated training chains are simply

overkill. These are for serious, competitive powerlifters, commercial gyms or home gym owners who want to hang their chains off bars next to the BMW or Audi.

Kettlebells

Kettlebells are not in the typical bodybuilder's arsenal of exercise weapons. For home gym bodybuilders, you may want to rethink this.

The versatility, price and footprint of kettlebells are hard to match. Let's see why.

First, because most kettlebell movements engage muscles in most of the body—full-body movements—they represent an excellent method for warming up, to prime the pump and grease the basic movements, for the typical hypertrophy training to follow. The value of this cannot be underestimated. Think about all the days when you got up, or got home from work, and just didn't feel like working out (that can also be an indicator of insufficient recovery, but that's a story for another day). Now, think about those times where you eventually did drag yourself into the gym and started moving working out. You started to feel better and may have had a productive training session. Warming up with kettlebells is a great method to warm-up both physically and mentally for the work ahead. In mere minutes, you can open the hips, warm the core and get your heart pounding. It's a nice gradual elevation of the mental and physical preparedness necessary for progress.

Second, kettlebells are an effective aid in hypertrophy training and for direct cardio work. Let's take the cardio first. Several studies have demonstrated that a 20-minute kettlebell snatch workout burns about 13 calories per minute, *during the entire workout*. That's the equivalent to running at a 6-minute per mile pace. Topping that off, as an adjunct to hypertrophy training, lateral raises, abdominal movements, upright rows with kettlebells are hard to beat.

Third, because you only need a few weight increments here, these things are relatively inexpensive. At minimum, you can start with one. At most, three to four weight increment pairs are all you'll need.

Fourth, they are portable. If you are one of those guys (or gals) that have a compulsive urge to work out on vacation, then take a kettlebell. If you like to do your cardio outside, then take a kettlebell and add some anaerobic work to the workout.

Finally, because you don't need many of these, they don't take up much space. Think about that—a cardio and hypertrophy aid (not to mention power and endurance), combined into a few kettlebells that probably occupy about two square feet of your home gym. This is where Dan John says, "The [kettlebell] swing is a fat-burning athlete builder". It builds bodybuilders too. That's a win all the way around. In addition, they are an excellent way to introduce kids and other novices to conditioning, flexibility, hypertrophy and the whole wonderful world of weight training.

Kettlebells vs. Dumbbells

If you've already got adjustable or fixed dumbbells, you may be thinking you don't need any kettlebells, right? Maybe. Technically, you can do all the kettlebell moves with a dumbbell—swings, Turkish getups, etc,--but they're kind of awkward and not as effective. Here's why.

The main difference, besides thickness of the handle, is how the load is balanced. Kettlebells are designed to throw you off-balance, because they are not balanced like a dumbbell. As you lift, your body is constantly working to fight the off-balance aspect. Therefore, in general, kettlebell work is more difficult than a dumbbell at the same weight. The only direct equivalency is the weight stamped on each.

Bottom line—kettlebells aren't dumbbells and dumbbells are not kettebells. Use each appropriately.

Budget Kettlebells ($10-$20)
Make yourself two kettlebells—one for lower body movements and a lighter one for overhead movements and presses. An old basketball, some

quick drying cement and PVC are all you need. The Internet is full of DIY kettlebell plans, but they all boil down to those three ingredients.

Economy Kettlebells ($50-$100)

Get two pairs of kettlebells (one for lower body, another for swings and presses), used is fine—although Amazon sells new ones for reasonable prices with free shipping.

Luxury Kettlebells ($250+)

Buy a series of kettlebells at various weights or opt for a set of cast-iron adjustable bells.

Wrist Rollers

Strong forearms and grip strength are essential to weight training. Normal, progressive resistance training with exercises that require grip strength, such as deadlifts and shrugs should develop this naturally. However, for those seeking additional, focused development in this area, a wrist roller can be an effective adjunct to this training.

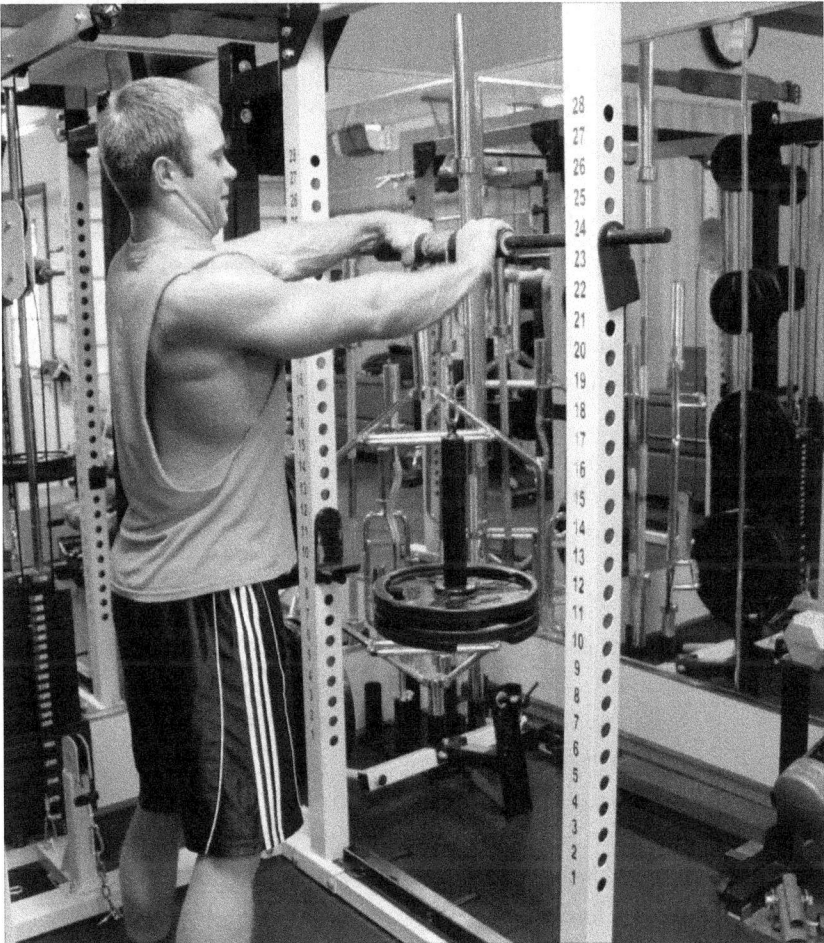

You have two effective options here. Obtain a thick bar wrist roller, such as that sold by IronMind, or build a wrist rolling station on your power rack. I like this latter option because it provides both the equipment and the most effective setup for executing the action. It's also cheap (the wrist roller slides right over the safety rod—you did get rods on your power rack, didn't you?), so a win for us all around.

DIY Wrist Roller

You'll need a length of 1.5" PVC pipe, a dog leash and some double-sided electrical tape. The general idea here is to cut the PVC to slide over the power rack's spotting rod (hopefully your rack uses rods, otherwise you're down to the handheld IronMind option), so cut the PVC to fit the rod's length inside the cage. The PVC acts as a bushing, allowing everything to turn smoothly. Attach the dog collar to the PVC and wrap as much electrical tape as you feel is necessary around the pipe.

When you are ready to do some wrist rolling, just slide your DIY wrist roller over the spotting rod, set the rod at shoulder height and attach a weight to the end of the dog collar. Stand back a bit, keep your arms straight and start turning the roller to lift the weight. If you think rolling the weight all the way up is challenging, the controlled journey down can be just as bad.

Budget Wrist Roller ($5)
Use the plan above and build one yourself in about ten minutes for a fiver.

Economy Wrist Roller ($15-$25)
You can buy standard issue wrist rollers at most sporting goods stores or major Internet retailers. They won't be thick bar or might not be knurled, but then you get what you pay for.

Luxury Wrist Roller ($35-$70)
The difference here is knurling and girth. Luxury, heavy-duty wrist rollers are 2" thick bars with heavy knurling. They will hold any load you can put on them and will last forever although your forearms will think they are dying.

Foam Rollers & Other Self-Healing Tools

Implementing soft tissue foam rolling into your training is an effective, inexpensive way to increase mobility and performance, prevent injuries and help to assist in reducing or eliminating many muscle imbalances. All this for about $40 and 5-10 minutes per day.

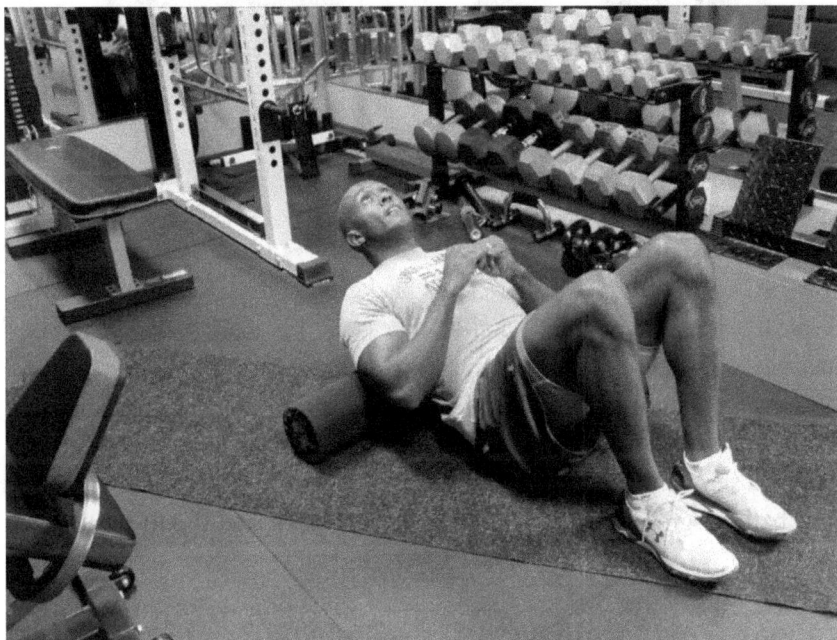

Unlike pre-workout static and dynamic stretching, foam rolling has no negative effects on performance—it increases range of motion without decreasing muscle activation or force. Foam rolling mimics myofascial release techniques and is a lot cheaper than occasional visits to the chiropractor. Therefore, foam rolling is good for our bodybuilding efforts and we should use it, especially given the low investment cost.

If you don't have a good foam roller—or even if you do—rolling on tennis, lacrosse, and golf balls works well and provides even finer targeted myofascial release.

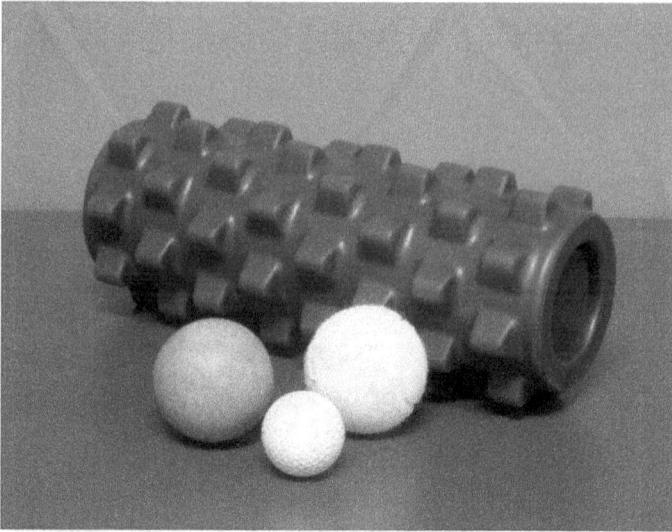

Budget Foam Roller ($0)

For those coming from an experienced background in foam rolling, you can use a barbell loaded with smaller plates (the 10s work well here). I say experienced, because the barbell variety of myofascial rolling provides an intense, targeted release, due to the small diameter of the bar. Think of the difference between a typical 5" diameter foam roller and a barbell as that between a shotgun and a laser. For others on a budget, try rolling with a tennis ball, progressing to a lacrosse ball and finally, a golf ball for targeted precision.

Economy Foam Roller ($10)

Get a piece of PVC pipe (try a 5" diameter first) that is 36" long. PVC is hard as hell, but works. If the PVC is too hard for you, try wrapping a towel or carpet remnant around the pipe and securing it with duct tape.

Luxury Foam Roller ($40-$70)

Dedicated, commercial foam rollers are available just about everywhere these days. Beware of those that emphasize padding and comfort—that may feel good in the beginning, but will minimize effectiveness quickly as your body adapts. Stick with ones that are 36" long and 5" in diameter.

Ab Mat

Now, before you think I've exceeded my scope by recommending superfluous pieces of fitness gear, there are two specific areas where an ab mat can make a huge impact—Gironda-style sit-ups and lying leg curls.

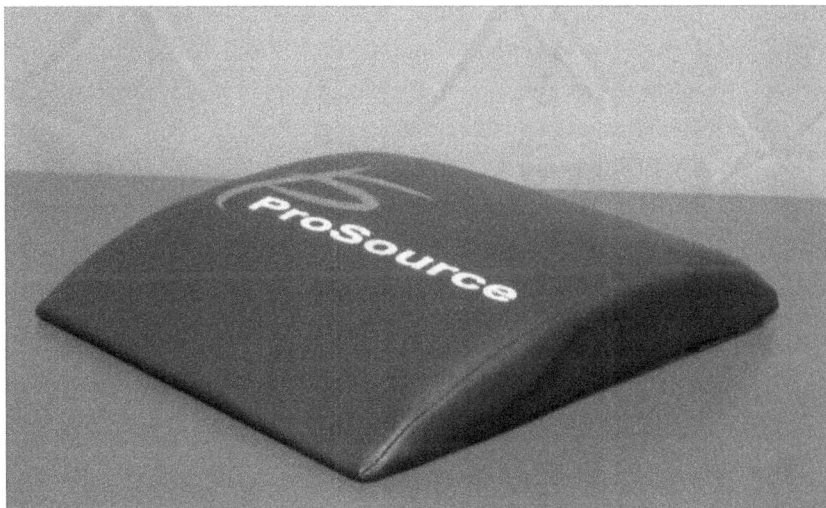

Gironda Sit-Ups with an Ab Mat

If you're not familiar with Gironda-style sit-ups (also called frog sit-ups), here's a brief synopsis of how they work.

Lie on the floor, flat on your back and place your heels up as close to your buttocks as possible. Spread your legs wide, like a frog. Now, curl your upper torso toward your midsection. This movement does a good job of isolating the abdominals and reducing involvement of the psoas and other related hip muscles.

By using an ab mat with this exercise, the range of motion is increased, stress on the lower back decreases, and results are improved.

Enhancing Lying Leg Curls with an Ab Mat

For those of you who opted for the lying leg curl attachment for your adjustable bench (I'm including myself here), you may have noticed why some commercial lying leg curl machines are so much more safe and effective—the bench you lie on is angled so that the spine is opened up while under load. This is not the case with leg curl attachments. The flat bench surface can cause lower back impingement as the load increases or execution form starts breaking down. By placing an ab mat at the lower end of your bench, just above where the leg curl attaches, you can gain some of the benefits of an angled commercial leg curl unit. I say some, because the ab mat does not provide the extreme angle that those machines typically offer. However, it does increase safety and force transfer, so spending $20-$30 here can benefit both your abs and your hamstrings. To me, that's worth it.

Barbell Pad

Typically, you see novice (or experienced—but still novice!) weight trainers using a barbell pad for cushioning of the bar against the upper back and traps. I don't advocate a bar pad for that use, because it tends to create an unstable environment for a loaded bar. Your upper back and traps can hold the bar much more effectively on their own. Remember, exercise is not comfortable. You don't produce a systemic change with comfort.

What a bar pad is really useful for is to minimize the pain associated with the bar directly contacting bone, such as your elbows and knees when performing Zercher squats or with seated calf raises. So, if comfort here is important to you (and bone bruising is not), then spending about $20 for a barbell pad may be worth it. Otherwise, rolled up towels will work in a pinch.

Suspension Trainers

German gymnasts and schoolchildren first began using suspended rings (*ringeschwebel*) in the 1800s as a method of fitness conditioning. I only advocate the use of a suspension-training device for a finishing move with bodybuilding-type work, because it's almost impossible to accurately and consistently regulate the load with these types of body weight movements.

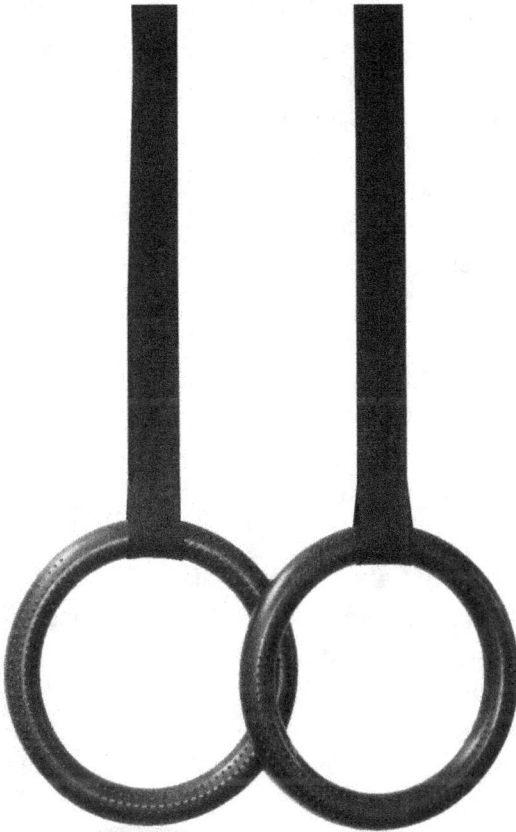

I was skeptical of suspension training until I conjured up my variety of Vince Gironda's famous hanging rings, and tried Mr. Olympia Larry Scott's version of flies using these things. Somehow, dumbbell flies seem far easier and less effective after performing flies with a suspension trainer. What else can you use these suspension trainers for? How about finishing your workout with pull-ups or chin-ups? In many cases, they tend to be kinder to your elbows than a straight chinning bar.

Here then are the advantages of suspension training devices:

- They are quick to hook up to a power rack or basement rafters.

- They are an effective tool for beginners through profession athletes.

- They develop balance, strengthen the core, muscles and joints. Additionally, they work the stabilizer muscles that you didn't even know you had more effectively that almost anything else.

And I've mentioned the big disadvantage:

- They use gravity, your body weight and leverage (incline and decline your body to increase or decrease the intensity). This is hard to quantify in absolute numbers for tracking purposes.

Suspensions trainers should be one of the last things you obtain for your home gym, given the long-term effectiveness of the dumbbells and barbells. They are icing on the cake.

Books & Videos

Noted brain surgeon Ben Carson has continually emphasized the importance of reading as a prime method of exercising the mind. In fact, he states "reading does activate the mind in the same way that we activate muscles when we lift weights."

Many of us who train with weights recognize this. The problem is the type of source material most select—and most select magazines, like *Muscle & Fitness*, *Flex*, etc. There are two problems here. First, most of these magazines feature drug-laden bodybuilders with workout routines that require performance-enhancing drugs (steroids) for recovery. Second, these magazines are expensive, when you consider the price you pay for original, quality information per page. I remember years ago, when my memory was still razor sharp, reading an article in *Muscle & Fitness* that seemed strangely familiar. Sure enough, after digging through my cache of old issues, I found *the exact same article, word for word*, except this time attributed to a different "author" and with different pictures.

Once you come to grips with the fact that professional writers pen these articles and not bodybuilders—that the article content is regurgitated every couple of years in their entirety, and that they rarely provide any deviation from volume-based training dogma (but they do sell fairly useless supplements!), you start to realize the importance of good weight training books.

The lesson here is to spend your money on quality books to both broaden and deepen your understanding of how to maximize muscular growth. In the end, it's going to save you a lot of money.

Essential (Classic) Books

Hundreds of good bodybuilding books are available. However, it's the rare few, which communicate essential concepts clearly, broaden our knowledge and become classics. I recommend you buy each of the classic books listed below. Read and absorb the knowledge within and you'll know more than just about anyone in any gym.

Bill Pearl's Keys to the Inner Universe

Although many consider Arnold's book (see below) as the bible of bodybuilding, Pearl's equally massive tome has something that even Arnold didn't produce—over 700 barbell, dumbbell and cable exercises and variations you can perform. That is a godsend for the home gym bodybuilder who plans to train with a few pieces of equipment for years. In addition, lots of good routines for the drug-free bodybuilder.

Arnold Schwarzenneger's Encyclopedia of Modern Bodybuilding

This book covers all the basics of volume-based training, dieting, contest prep, etc. Every aspiring bodybuilder should have this book.

The Complete Keys to Progress

In this book from John McCallum, you can follow the weightlifting adventures of Ollie, Marvin, and Uncle Harry. Although the stories hold your attention, the lessons are the bedrock of any type of weight training.

The Strongest Shall Survive

Although the subtitle is *Strength Training for Football*, you can largely ignore that. Here, legendary strength coach Bill Starr lays out the foundation for strength and hypertrophy correctly. This book inspired a young Mark Rippetoe.

Starting Strength: Basic Barbell Training

Here, noted strength coach Mark Rippetoe breaks down the essential of barbell training in exquisite detail. If longevity in lifting, minimizing the risk of injury, and maximizing muscular adaptation is important to you, you'll get this book.

Other Good Books

Bodybuilding: A Scientific Approach

Written by powerlifting god and guru Dr. Fred Hatfield ('Dr. Squat'), this book exposes you to holistic training, aimed at maximizing muscular growth based on muscle fiber type.

Brawn

Any of the books in the Brawn series by Stuart McRobert are worthwhile reading. Start with the first book, which lays the foundation.

Loaded Guns

Here, the first Mr. Olympia Larry Scott proves he didn't just know arm training. Filled with all the little details of exercise performance—which can make a drastic improvement in your results. Lots of stuff here originated with Vince Gironda, one of Larry's trainers.

Brother Iron, Sister Steel

This book is worth it, just to absorb the passion, love, and longevity of lifting from Mr. Universe Dave Draper ('The Blonde Bomber'). It doesn't hurt that it's also filled with nuggets of useful info that's hard to find anywhere else, especially because Dave's been doing this for over 60 years.

Championship Bodybuilding

Chris Aceto is well known in the professional bodybuilding circuit for his contest prep work in diet and training. In this book, Chris details specific aspects of hypertrophy training that can elevate your results from mediocre to exceptional.

Sliced

In bodybuilding, it's not all about the training. Diet is equally important and this book details the ins and outs of performance nutrition, so you can keep that hard-earned muscle while stripping away the fat. It's also got the best visual descriptions of varying levels of body fat that I've ever seen.

Ripped

Clarence Bass ushered in the era of ultra-lean physiques with his performance in the Mr. America contests of the 1970s (over 40 age bracket). His Ripped series of books lays out the plans he followed in both training and diet to achieve this conditioning. They are based on sound, scientific and meticulous concepts.

Stretching

The importance of training for flexibility cannot be underestimated—it can have a significant effect on developing your muscular potential. This 1970s book is still the definitive guide to stretching.

Videos

Books can tell you a lot, but they can't show you everything. That's where training videos come in.

Sometimes you need a video to understand the intricacies of a particular exercise's performance. Or, you might require one to motivate you after a long day at work. Thanks to the Internet, you don't have to pay for most of this. YouTube is full of free training, instructional and motivational videos, seminars and documentaries about weight training and bodybuilding. Although you may have to sift through a lot of junk to find the good stuff, the good stuff is generally very good. If you don't know where to start, begin with Mark Rippetoe's *Strarting Strength* channel on YouTube. He has dozens of training videos, interviews, and seminars available for free. I downloaded his entire library onto a USB stick, which I have plugged into my SmartTV that hangs in my home gym. Instant motivation, inspiration and instruction. For pure natural bodybuilding, five-time Mr. Universe Skip La Cour offers reasonably priced training and instructional videos in various formats. ExRx.net is another free site that offers hundreds of instructional exercise videos, along with training plans and general physiology information.

Watch a video to get your head in the game, as coach would say, then put on some music to get in the combat-ready zone.

Heart Rate Monitor

Heart Rate Monitors (HRMs) provide an objective method of measuring your conditioning (cardio) work, allowing you to document progress and improvement. Effectively, they allow you to program your conditioning work over time.

Marty Gallagher is a big proponent of incorporating a heart rate monitor into conditioning work and so am I. But you say your exercise bike, treadmill or elliptical already has one built-in. Yes, but lots of people bought cars with integrated phones and antennas back in the 1990s, until they realized they needed the phone when they were driving *another car*. Same argument here. What if you suddenly get the urge to go for a trail walk, jog through the neighborhood or god forbid, actually ride a bike down the street?

This is where the versatility of strapping on one of these devices becomes evident.

Now, although we can debate the accuracy of the built-in heart monitors within various pieces of cardio equipment, their accuracy is easily eclipsed by any heart rate monitor that includes a chest strap.

Here are the base features your heart rate monitor needs:

- Average Heart Rate
- Max Heart Rate
- Target Zone
- Time in Target Zone

Two final notes here. HRMs are particularly effective when using more than one type of cardio training—which is something all of us should be doing ('everything works for about six weeks, nothing works forever'). In addition, if you are using kettlebell training for conditioning work, you might not want to use the monitor, because those kettlebells will be interacting with your forearm and wrist extensively. A game of rock, paper, scissors with cast iron and electronics has a clear winner.

Budget Heart Rate Monitor ($60)
Just the basic tracking we need to get the job done effectively and efficiently.

Economy Heart Rate Monitor ($90)
Adds auditory cues when you enter and leave your THR zone—which is nice so you don't fall or crash your bike while looking at the watch.

Luxury Heart Rate Monitor ($100+)
Adds the ability to do data transfer for record keeping. And we all keep records, don't we?

Hand-Grip Dynamometer

A what? One of the most effective methods for determining if you are over-reaching or have over-trained is to test grip strength. Here, we need an objective measure of grip strength—which means that simple grippers or even Captains of Crush™ are not useful. Handgrip dynamometers provide an integer-based objective result—something that you can record and track.

Here's the important part—never change the testing protocol.

Test your grip at the same time every day, with the same hand in the same posture, and same pre-test conditions (warmed up or going in cold). Then, do only one test and record the results.

With normal training recovery, there will be little daily variance in your grip (maybe 2-4 pounds). Insufficient recovery, fatigue or some disturbance in the force is indicated by variances greater than this. The greater the variance the more likely you have gone from over-reaching to over-training. This quick analysis allows you to make training program adjustments before issues arise. It allows you even more control.

I suggest using the classic Japanese production method for adjusting for variance. Don't make adjustments based on a single daily reading. Instead, if you see a downward trend lasting for several days—which is then considered a significant variance, then make an adjustment by reducing intensity and volume. Otherwise, you are just trying to herd sheep, which we all know is difficult unless you have a Border Collie.

Therefore, based on the effectiveness of this simple test, combined with a low price (about $30) for the device itself, this tool should be in every serious trainer's collection, regardless of activity. You can find these at online retailers. You won't find them at Walmart or mass market sporting goods chains.

Strive to keep your grip strength steady.

Video Camera & Tripod

Recording yourself performing an exercise movement is an excellent method to identify weaknesses. Because most of us have smartphones with built-in cameras that record video, the only thing missing is a tripod. Mounting your cellphone on a tripod in your home gym and recording video of yourself performing various movements is one of the best tools in your bag for detecting performance issues, muscle imbalances, and correcting them before injury results. You correct them by comparing your video against reputable videos of experts performing the same movement.

Make sure to get a full-height tripod used for cameras. You may also need a cellphone mount. This should set you back only about $20-$40, but that's much cheaper than a visit to the doctor or chiropractor.

Plastic Bins

Whatever accessory equipment you accumulate, having one or more plastic bins to hold things like belts, straps, foam rollers, spring clips, etc. keeps things organized and safely out of the way when you aren't using it. Even sturdy cardboard boxes will work. These things are cheap so get some.

Stuff You Don't Need

If you've spent any amount of time in a commercial gym, you'll see people wearing enough weightlifting accoutrements that it seems they are gearing up for battle. Gloves, belts, straps and wraps. We've talked about the usefulness of a belt and straps, but those other things—the gloves and wraps, in particular are not necessary, and can even sabotage your progress. Let me explain.

Gloves add a layer of unstable material between your God-given hands and the bar, dumbbell or handle you are gripping. This actually destabilizes the grip and can make gripping harder because you are effectively increasing the diameter of the thing being held (if that's what you are trying to do, there are better alternatives here, such as Fat Gripz™).

Knee and elbow wraps are useful if you are injured or training for a powerlifting meet—but because this book is about bodybuilding training, using wraps only allows you to fool yourself into thinking you can press and squat this way. We aren't interested in the stretch reflex they provide and the weaknesses they can hide.

Maintaining Your Equipment

The good news is that you now own your own gym and equipment. The bad news is that you just became your own janitor. (If you have kids, this is also an opportunity for a teaching experience on proper maintenance and cleaning. You see, there are carryover effects from the gym throughout most aspects of life.) Home gyms, like every other thing in your home, require cleaning and maintenance. I'll leave the cleaning details to you, but equipment checks are a must to ensure safety and effectiveness.

Things you will need to check periodically:

- **Bars**—check the sleeve rotation and tightness, clean the knurls with a wire brush and inspect the overall finish for any signs of oxidation and rust (chalk powder and sweat contribute to rust)—this is where dehumidifiers pay for themselves if you are training in a moist environment, such as unfinished basements or garages. If you need to oil your bars (use a light coat of 3-In-One or CLP oil) make sure to wipe them down afterwards. I've seen plates slide off the sleeves after a good oiling like they were skiing down Everest.

- **Cables**—check them for any sign of frays. If you see a cable starting to fray apart, replace it as soon as possible. In the meantime, *don't use it*. Years ago, at a small commercial gym I was training at, I watched a pulldown cable slowly fray apart over the course of several weeks. The inexperienced (or just plain stupid) owner used duct tape around the fraying cable in his attempt to 'fix' the problem. Now, I know duct tape works wonders and solves many problems on both Earth and in space (ask the Apollo 13 astronauts), but I didn't think it would hold together a cable supporting upwards of 300lbs (the capacity of that weight stack) and the accelerant force provided by the user. It didn't and the victim in the ensuing incident severely injured himself—not from the force of the bar slamming into his chest (which it did)—but from the twisting of his torso when he fell backward as his legs remained pinned under the thigh pads. I recorded a large mental and another gym lesson that day.

- **Bolts and Screws**—check all apparatus bolted or screwed together (benches, racks) for tightness. It can be amazing how quickly that bolt you tightened last month loosened slightly after several sessions of squats, presses and shrugs.

- **Welds**—after checking and tightening any bolts and screws on your equipment, check all welds to make sure they are free of cracking.

- **Collars and Clamps**—you check these every time you use them, don't you? If not, start doing it. An oversight here can be quite costly, especially with exercises where the weight is over your head. And yes, I've seen plates come off adjustable dumbbells during pullovers and hit people smack in the face. After 25 years in gyms, I've just about seen it all. Stupidity and lack of safety often result in injury, some of which can end your weightlifting career and alter your course in life.

- **Mirrors**—make sure they are clean and free of cracks. Try to use an ammonia-free cleaner instead of Windex. Little known fact—the ammonia in Windex eventually causes mirrors to deteriorate. The symptom is tiny black dots on the mirror. Next time you visit a hotel, check the mirrors for these imperfections. Of course, if you are using a $10 Walmart closest mirror, this really doesn't matter, does it?

- **Flooring**—just make sure the floor is clean, dry and has no slippery surface area.

I recommend performing these equipment checks at least quarterly—more frequently (monthly) if others use the gym as well.

8

Adding It All Up: What's It Gonna Cost?

Again, the answer here is—it depends. It depends on each decision you make regarding the room environment and equipment. Here are some ideas for how to stock your home gym at various price points. Remember, the goal here is bodybuilding, so the tools reflect that combination that will provide muscle hypertrophy along with a reduction in body fat. Remember, you can add equipment gradually as you get the funds.

Home Gym for Under $100

The key here is searching for great deals on used equipment.

- Two used adjustable plate-loaded dumbbells (with plates)
- Jump rope (but don't forget about walking outside)

Home Gym for $100-$250

Same as above, but we add a used adjustable bench and some solid flooring.

- Two used adjustable plate-loaded dumbbells (with plates)
- Used adjustable bench
- Jump rope
- One horse stall mat

Home Gym for Under $500

With $500, we can add the barbell and plates—and the mirror.

- Two used adjustable plate-loaded dumbbells (with plates)
- Used adjustable bench
- Used barbell and plates
- Jump rope
- Ab roller (come on, it's only $10)
- Two horse stall mats
- Cheap, closet-style mirror

Home Gym for Under $1000

For less than $1000, you can assemble the complete core experience for bodybuilding, including the all-important power rack, which unleashes your potential.

- Two used adjustable plate-loaded dumbbells (with plates)
- Used adjustable bench
- Used barbell and plates
- Power rack
- Used exercise bike
- Ab roller (come on, it's only $10)
- Two horse stall mats
- Two full-width closet mirrors

Core Equipment

Now, let's add up everything from the previous chapters, focusing on the core equipment. After each item, I'll list the budget, economy and luxury prices in parenthesis for quick reference. Where I've indicated ranges in the text, I'll take the average and list it here. For the plates, I'll use my prior recommendations of 175lbs in plates for novices, and 600lbs for everybody else. Couple that with used versus new prices per pound of plate, and that gives us a range for each budget category.

	Budget	Economy	Luxury
Dumbbells	$50	$200	$500
Adjustable Bench	$50	$100	$300
Barbell	$50	$100	$300
Plates	$90 to $225	$175 to $600	$300-$900
Rack	$250	$500	$1000
Flooring	$0	$70	$200
Total	**$500 to $650**	**$1000 to $1500**	**$2500 to $3500**

Once you have the core equipment in place, you can start adding a cable system and various accessory items, as described earlier as your space and budget allows.

Home Gym Checklist

I love checklists. They are useful for your training and your life, for organization and execution. You can use the following checklist as both a process and a reference for building out your home gym. Just mark off the things you already have, and then proceed to acquire or build additional items as your needs and budget dictate.

- ❑ Dumbbells
- ❑ Plates
- ❑ Adjustable Bench
- ❑ Barbell
- ❑ EZ Curl Bar
- ❑ Triceps Bar
- ❑ Hex Bar
- ❑ Barbell Collars
- ❑ Power Rack
- ❑ Leg Extension
- ❑ Leg Curl
- ❑ Cable System (high, low)
- ❑ Cable Attachments
- ❑ Cardio Equipment
- ❑ Training Journal
- ❑ Ab Wheel
- ❑ Foam Roller

If You Build It, Will You (They) Come?

Here's the key. Once you establish your home gym as a place that generates results, word will spread (after all, you become a walking physical advertisement of the results) and others will inevitably want to join in. This is a good thing.

As former National Champion Olympic Weightlifter Tommy Suggs would testify, training partners with similar interest and enthusiasm are almost as important as the equipment. It can magnify the training and the results. Tommy calls this the 'X-Factor', where individual enthusiasm, attitudes of success and yes—large egos combine to form a synergistic environment geared to progress. If you create something that is so compelling, you shouldn't have any problem attracting reliable lifting partners. This is pure gold.

Home gyms are not vast expanses of space and equipment. Use this to your advantage—lifting with workout partners in close quarters forces attentiveness and focus. It also tends to foster spotting, encouragement and coaching (on form, workout feedback, etc.). Everyone gets involved in each other's workout and it builds camaraderie and teamwork, something that was common in the Golden Age of bodybuilding in Venice, California at the original Gold's Gym in the 1960s and 1970s. You can recreate this to a large part in your facility.

After the workout is over, you've got a place to talk, eat, etc. This is how you generate ideas for future workouts and learn a lot of information. Jim Wendler likens this to the male version of the beauty salon.

The maximum capacity in most garage gyms is about four to six—for spare rooms it may be two—for basements maybe many more, and for outside structures and sheds—we'll that's dictated by the size of the structure. Got a barn—invite half of your old gym—the good half.

However, just like in kindergarten, if you are going to play with others you need some rules. Although you know what you expect, others may not, so it's best to communicate these expectations directly. Enter the gym rules.

Your Gym, Your Rules

This is your gym. You set the rules. Here are some suggestions—you'll find they are often the antithesis of the modern politically-correct, corporate, chain spa-gym. However, these types of rules foster an environment of safety, respect, camaraderie and results.

Here are some rules that should be common to all home gyms:

Gym Rules
Use Chalk
Load Music Only
Work Hard or Go Home
Grunting Allowed
Put Weights Away When Done
Break Your PRs
Train, Do Not Work Out
Respect the Equipment

One final point. Invite others to train with you, but don't charge them. That invites all kinds of legal issues if someone gets injured.

My Gym: One Man's Story

Many readers may be interested to see what I decided to put into my home gym. Remember, this is one man's story, based on the needs and goals of my family and me. Your results may vary. That's ok. I've mentioned some of my equipment throughout the book, but here it is in full.

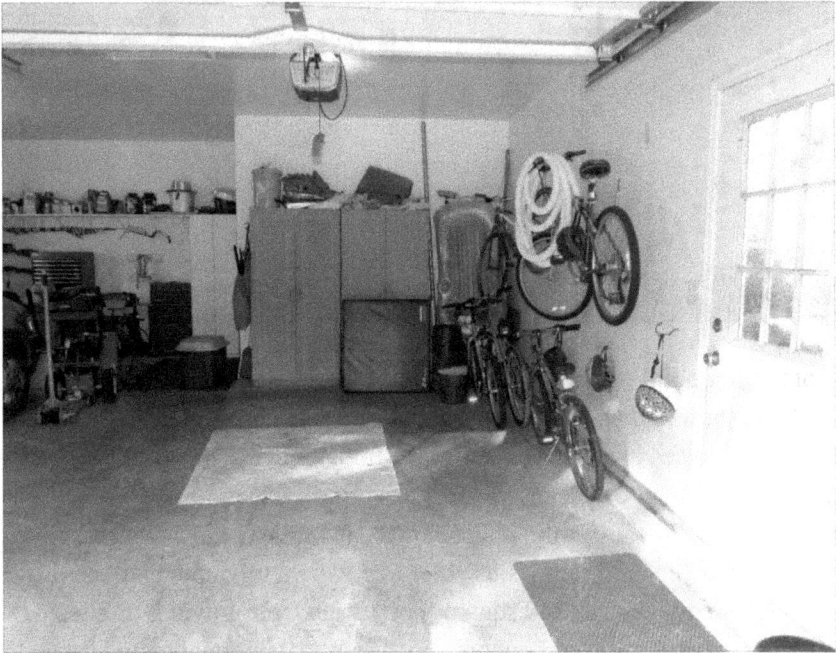

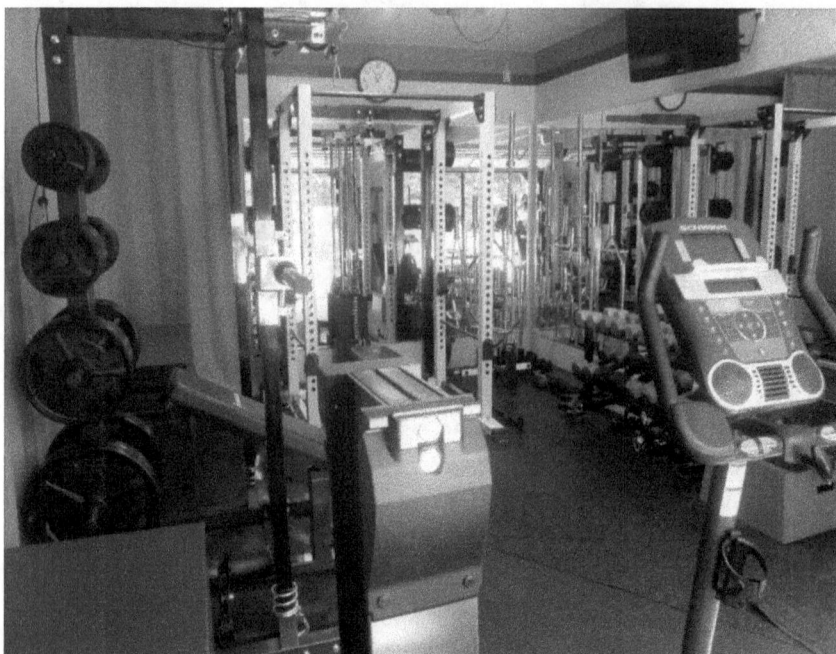

A continuing point—I did not acquire this "stuff" en masse. It was purchased (new and used), traded for, and in some cases, given by friends and acquaintances over the years. From a bodybuilder's perspective, there is nary a movement or exercise I can't perform in this gym. We've regularly had six of us training here at the same time (I have two racks—my Smith Machine also allows use of a free weight Olympic bar—so this is doable), so my meager 240 square foot garage gym provides all the inspiration, perspiration and opportunity as any commercial gym. Use this as incentive for your own setup.

The Room

12'x20' garage (one-half of a two-car garage) with a 9' ceiling.

The Floor

Cement, covered completely with ten ¾" thick horse stall mats.

Lighting

Two 4' banks of fluorescent lights (4 bulbs each, 8 total)

Mirrors

Two walls of 6' tall commercial mirrors, providing 25 feet of mirror length

Climate Control

- Electric forced-air space heater in the winter
- 24" industrial fan and 14,000 BTU portable air conditioner/dehumidifier in the summer

Sound & Video

- Portable stereo with radio and iPod dock.
- Wall mounted Internet-connected 32" Smart TV.

Dumbbells

- 5-50lb fixed, cast-iron dumbbells in 5lb increments (2.5lb increments with PlateMates™)
- 10-120lb cast iron adjustable dumbbells in 2.5lb increments

Plates

- 1000lbs of rubberized cast-iron plates in 5, 10, 25, and 45lb sizes
- Two 1.25lb cast-iron micro-loading plates

Benches

- Flat Utility Bench
- Adjustable Bench (flat, incline, decline)

Barbells

- 7' Olympic bar
- 5' Olympic bar
- E-Z Curl bar
- Triceps bar
- Trap bar

Racks

Full-size 84" tall power rack with 300lb weight stack and high/ low cables, chin and dip bars.

Machines

- Leg Extension/Curl attachment
- Preacher/Spider Curl attachment
- Vertical Leg Press
- Smith Machine with high/ low cables, adjustable width chin bar

Cardio Equipment

- Stationary bike
- Concept 2 rower
- Jump ropes

Accessories

- Ab wheel
- Ab pad
- Calf block
- Chalk
- Dip belt
- Landmine
- Two 12" high plyometric boxes
- Four cast-iron fixed weight kettlebells (15lbs, 20lbs)
- Two adjustable cast-iron kettlebells (25-80lbs)
- Two foam rollers
- Various cable attachments
- Wrist roller with vertical plate loading pin

Inspiration, Perspiration and Desire

In the end, it's the man and his effort, not the location or equipment, which matters most. It's the gestalt of all that stuff you acquired and put in place that hopefully ignites, fuels and continues to burn the desire, determination and true grit that will make all the difference.

Don't forget—you're supposed to enjoy your training. Maybe not all the time, or even when you are smack in the belly of the beast. Nevertheless, you should be able to look back at your training sessions and have a deep sense of accomplishment, fulfillment, gratitude and purpose. Otherwise, what's the point? Surrounding yourself with the equipment and environment that supports this enjoyment is paramount. If you follow the steps and guidance in this book, you'll have everything you need to train like a bodybuilder for the rest of your life. But will you?

Over time, inspiration and desire may shift with your needs and goals. Consequently, your home gym will evolve to meet those needs. Stuff that was important in the past may be less so as you age. Other things may move to the forefront. Mobility and strength have a lifecycle requiring changes in methods and priorities. Change is not to be feared, but embraced through thought, planning and execution.

• • • •

It's on those coldest of winter's solitary nights, as you determine how and why you will try to push that bar away from Earth's grip for yet another rep, that you discover the essence of your character. Like the answer or not, it's all you. You alone determine your destiny and how you will face it. In the end, little has changed in a million years.

9

Beyond the Home Gym

The home gym blueprints here extend to the commercial gym setting as well. Many have built a home gym with aspirations limited to just training at home, but eventually grew that gym into a successful commercial enterprise, whether for personal training, coaching, full-blown gym or fitness center. However, most of us will remain with our home gyms—hopefully, training for as long as God allows.

If you do decide to train others in your home gym, especially in exchange for money, I urge you to investigate and educate yourself about liability and local small business law. The first step here is to find out if you are even able to train people and charge money at your location. Many homeowner's associations, rental agreements, and local jurisdiction property law prohibit it. Additionally, it's best to be prepared for worst case scenarios, in case someone does get injured in spite of your diligence for safety. Lifting heavy things is inherently dangerous.

Leaving the Gym at the Gym

Your training and your physique does not define you and it shouldn't consume you. It's one part of you. Family, friends, relationships and your interaction with them defines you. I talked about this in my earlier book, *Supermen: Building Maximum Muscle for a Lifetime*, and it's an important point I want you to always keep in mind.

I am far from alone in this view. Here are two examples.

In 1992, I attended the Arnold Classic bodybuilding competition in Columbus, Ohio. There were many speakers during the weekend, but the one I remember most was the legendary bodybuilder, Reg Park, also famous for his many Hercules movies in the 1950s and 1960s. Although all the other speakers talked about the intricacies or simplicities of training and nutrition, Reg wanted to talk about *not training*. Specifically, he talked about keeping your life in balance, not allowing bodybuilding to consume your life, especially at the expense of friends and family.

In a similar vein, strength coach Dan John stresses the importance of core values, and where your training should fit within a life balance of friends, family and faith.

These are important concepts to embody, in order to live a truly full life, one that you can be both proud and fulfilled to look back upon.

⑩

Beginner, Intermediate & Advanced Bodybuilding Workout Routines

Now that you've built the home gym, it's time to build you. If you have followed the suggestions in this book, your home gym will not equate to a second-rate workout. This section provides some well-tested bodybuilding training routines that have produced excellent results over the past decades. These systems are important to ensure intensity and transformation.

Beginner, intermediate or advanced? How do you know which stage you are? In many popular bodybuilder books and magazines, they typically use a general time-based estimate (0-6 month's beginner, 6 months-2 years intermediate, 2+ years advanced). This simplification generally holds true, because excellence demands time.

Additionally, because we are all descended from the same basic human genome, the beginner stage of progressive resistance adaptation holds true for just about all of us. It's the migration from intermediate to advanced where this all starts to break down. Most men and women who enter a gym, once past that beginner stage, never moves from the intermediate field of play. Why? They will say that they have "hit a plateau", "can't seem to improve" or that "nothing works". Well nothing always works— it's just that they don't have the knowledge, skill and—how should we say this—fortitude, to launch themselves into the advanced realm.

However, experience does not necessarily equate to skill or progression level. I know many people with 30+ years of driving experience, but I wouldn't call some of them 'advanced'.

This is where strength coach Mark Rippetoe's definitions become relevant.

Rippetoe's definition of a beginner, intermediate or advanced weight trainer is adaptation and results oriented. A beginner can increase their weights and improve from each workout, an intermediate generally requires a week's worth of structured workouts for improved results, and the advanced trainer must use periodization and planning to induce adaptations over a much longer period, often measured in months or years. Therein lies the rub—planning. Humans generally are not good at it, especially when it requires long-term planning, like mapping out an individualized weight lifting progression system over the course of a year. I'll give you some ideas on how to accomplish this below.

Before you leap into one of the routines below, let's make sure you understand some common principles and recommendations. For those of you who have been doing this weightlifting thing for some time now, I really shouldn't have to state these—but my eyes tell me I do every time I enter a gym.

General Bodybuilding Principles

Use a full range of motion. Half reps build half a physique.

Don't throw weights (momentum). You lift weights.

Use proper form. Do it and you're already in the minority.

If you feel pain when doing an exercise, then don't do it.

For more insights regarding bodybuilding training, you can refer to my book, *Supermen: Building Maximum Muscle for a Lifetime*.

Finally, a word about the workouts you'll find below.

If you see an exercise that you don't know or know how to do properly—and even if you do know—verify the correct performance again, and again. Use those book and video references I talked about earlier.

If you see an exercise in parenthesis immediately following another, that's an alternative movement that you can substitute in case you don't have the equipment or ability to perform that suggested exercise.

Let's go.

Beginning Bodybuilding

All of us are beginners at some point. If we're wise, intelligent or even lucky in our relationships, we can accumulate the knowledge and apply it—because, just like puberty, it's gonna be over real quick even if we don't think so while it's happening.

Beginners (novices) need to lay the foundation of strength, balance and mobility, upon which additional muscularity can be added. In this vein, the training is much like that of powerlifters, where the emphasis is on kinesthetic awareness—learning a limited set of basic compound movement patterns that involve as many muscles as possible, while adapting the central nervous system to hard work.

I recommend following an acclimation program for the first month. The purpose of this program is to learn the movement patterns of your starting set of exercises, using the equipment you acquired by following the strategy described earlier. I'll assume the minimal amount of equipment first, then subsequent beginner routines will expand on that as your equipment options grow. You'll also gradually acclimate your body to exercise variety, volume, intensity and hard work. This is the foundation the beginner needs in order to progress to the intermediate level.

The general novice bodybuilding strategy for progression is to start with full body workouts (three days per week), eventually progressing to a simple two-way split routine (upper/lower body). Launching directly into an intermediate-level five-way split routine is not the way forward for a novice, regardless of genetics, recovery ability or lack of intelligence.

Beginners may also want to keep these points in mind:

- If you've never lifted weights before, spend a week learning and getting used to the exercises before adding weight.

- Start lighter than you think you should. It's far better for long-term results to start light, slowly work your way up, learning the proper biomechanics of each movement. Bad form at the start will magnify as you add weight, which can result in injury or worse.

- The first several weeks shouldn't be that hard. As you near the one-month mark, struggles may start. This is normal. This is where perseverance, desire and intelligence combine to forge your future.

Full-Body Workout #1

🕒 *30-60 minutes (19-24 sets)*
⊤ *Dumbbells*

This is a complete hypertrophy-based program that requires three days per week, 30-60 minutes each session. It represents a full-body routine that works everything and is a good way to begin your bodybuilding and life-altering journey. Start with just the floor and a pair of dumbbells. Later, as you acquire more equipment, use a bench, a barbell and a rack to take this workout to new heights.

3 Days per Week

Exercise	Sets	Reps
Squats	3-4	15-20
Floor Press	3-4	8-12
Bent-Over or One-Arm Row	3-4	8-12
Lying Extensions	3-4	8-12
Curls	3-4	8-12
Reverse Crunches	2	To failure
Crunches	2	To failure

Full-Body Workout #2

🕐 *30-45 minutes (19 sets)*
🏋 *Dumbbells*

This workout is straightforward and focus-driven—ten exercises, each for
ten reps per set. Perform this low-volume, high-intensity workout three
days per week (how about the venerable Monday, Wednesday, and
Friday?). Make sure to do one or two light warm-up sets before each
working set listed below. Other than the first exercise, you'll be
performing two working sets of 10 reps for each exercise. After 6-8 weeks
on this program, take a week of rest, then move up to a more advanced
program.

3 Days per Week

Exercise	Sets	Reps
Side Bends	1	10
Squats	2	10
Stiff-Legged Deadlifts	2	10
Calf Raises	2	10
Floor Press	2	10
Bent-Over or One-Arm Rows	2	10
Standing Press	2	10
Curls	2	10
Lying Extensions	2	10
Sit-Ups	2	10

Full-Body Workout #3

🕐 30-45 minutes (13 sets)
Ⴤ Dumbbells and/or Barbell, Bench, Power Rack

This is a good introduction to the world of low-volume, high-intensity bodybuilding training. As indicated below, perform 1-2 working sets of each exercise for the prescribed number of reps (make sure you warm up with each exercise first—we don't count those warm-up sets). If you can't do 12 reps of the chin-up exercise listed below, substitute any other type of chins (such as Inverted Pull-Ups) you can do for 12 reps. Take 2-3 minutes rest between sets.

3 Days per Week

Exercise	Sets	Reps
Crunches	1	To failure
Squats	2	20
Stiff-Legged Deadlifts	1	10
Chins or Lat Pulldowns	1	12
Bench Press	2	6
Bent-Over Rows	2	8
Seated Press	1	6
Curls	1	6
Calf Raises	1	15
Crunches	1	To failure

Full-Body Workout #4

🕐 *20-60 minutes (12-24 sets)*
🍴 *Dumbbells, Barbell, Adjustable Bench, Power Rack*

This workout introduces you to a few exercises you may have never performed before. The first two weeks, perform one set of 10-12 reps on each exercise. For weeks 3-6, perform two sets of 10 reps for each. For the abdominal exercises, try to work up to 15-20 reps. Take 1-2 minutes rest between sets.

3 Days per Week

Exercise	Sets	Reps
Incline Press	1-2	10-12
One-Arm Row	1-2	10-12
Bent-Over Rear DB Laterals	1-2	10-12
Bench Dips	1-2	10-12
Curls	1-2	10-12
DB Side Laterals	1-2	10-12
Reverse Curls	1-2	10-12
Front Squats	1-2	10-12
Good Mornings	1-2	10-12
Calf Raises, One-Leg	1-2	10-12
Hanging Leg Raises, Bent-Knee	1-2	15-20
Sit-Ups	1-2	15-20

Full-Body Workout #5

⏲ 30-45 minutes (15-21 sets)
Ⳑ Barbell, Bench, Power Rack

This classic higher-rep, high-intensity workout starts by warming you up with lots of core exercises—then proceeds to one exercise for each major muscle group (make sure to warm-up on each of these subsequent exercises). Take 1-3 minutes rest between sets, as necessary.

3 Days per Week

Exercise	Sets	Reps
Sit-Ups	1	15-50
Side Bends	1	15-50
Alternating Leg Raises	1	15-50
Bench Press	2-3	10-15
Standing or Seated Press	2-3	10-15
Chins or Lat Pulldowns	2-3	10-15
Seated Extensions	2-3	10-15
Curls	2-3	10-15
Squats	2-3	10-15

Full-Body Workout #6

🕐 *30-45 minutes (16 sets)*
🍴 *Dumbbells, Barbell, Power Rack, High Cable*

This is full-body, high-intensity bodybuilding personified—you get only one shot at each exercise, so make it count. Unless otherwise directed, perform one set of each exercise for the prescribed number of reps (make sure you warm up with each exercise first—we don't count those warm-up sets). If you can't do 12 reps of the chin-up exercises listed below, substitute any other type of chins you can do for 12 reps.

3 Days per Week

Exercise	Sets	Reps
Squats	2	20
One-Leg DB Calf Raises	2	20 (each leg)
Standing or Seated Press	1	12
Rear Chins (Lat Pulldowns)	1	12
Bench Press	1	12
Bent-Over Rows	1	12
Pushdowns	1	12
Curls	1	12
Standing Extensions	1	12
Front Chins (Lat Pulldowns)	1	12
Pushdowns	1	12
Stiff-Legged Deadlifts	1	15
Wrist Curls	1	12
Crunches	1	12

Full-Body Workout #7

🕐 *45 minutes (20-21 sets)*
🍸 *Barbell, Bench, Power Rack*

Here's a low-variety, moderate-volume full-body workout, using the "Golden Six" exercises.

3 Days per Week

Exercise	Sets	Reps
Squats	4	10
Bench Press	3	10
Chin-Ups (Lat Pulldowns)	3	To failure
Standing or Seated Presses	4	10
Barbell Curls	3	10
Sit-Ups	3-4	To failure

Full-Body Workout #8

🕐 *60 minutes (42 sets)*
🍴 *Barbell, Bench, Power Rack*

This is a good workout to gauge how well your body handles and recovers from high volumes of work. Ten sets of each exercise with reps starting at ten and decreasing by one each set (10,9,8,7,6,5,4,3,2,1). Rest between sets should start at about one minute and decrease as the reps decrease—take more or less as you need it. Good luck.

3 Days per Week

Exercise	Sets	Reps
Front Squats	10	10, 9, 8, 7, 6, 5, 4, 3, 2, 1
Bench Press	10	10, 9, 8, 7, 6, 5, 4, 3, 2, 1
Chin-Ups (Lat Pulldowns)	10	10, 9, 8, 7, 6, 5, 4, 3, 2, 1
Deadlifts	10	10, 9, 8, 7, 6, 5, 4, 3, 2, 1
Crunches or Leg Raises	2	15

Full-Body Workout #9

🕐 *45-60 minutes (33 sets)*
🍸 *Dumbbells, Barbell, Bench, Power Rack*

Here is another classic full-body routine for those who have acclimated to high-volume training.

3 Days per Week

Exercise	Sets	Reps
Squats	3	7-10
Bench Press	3	7-10
DB Fly	3	7-10
DB Side Lateral Raise	3	7-10
Alternate DB Press	3	7-10
One-Arm DB Row	3	7-10
Barbell Curl	3	7-10
DB Concentration Curl	3	7-10
DB Wrist Curl	3	7-10
DB Side Bend	3	7-10
Sit-Ups	3	8-12

Full-Body 4-Month Program

🕐 *45-60 minutes*

Ⓨ *Dumbbells, Barbell, Power Rack, High Cable, Leg Extension/Curl*

If you are a novice trainer and are serious about packing on muscle, then this full body routine will get you where you want to go. You'll need to work out three days per week, for 45-60 minutes each session. The suggested workout days are Monday, Wednesday, and Friday, although you can change that to anything that fits your schedule—just try to keep one rest day between each workout. This is a four month program—just follow the workouts below for the weeks indicated. As you progress, the volume of work and exercise variety increases, building a solid foundation of movement, strength, muscle and overall conditioning. For the first couple weeks, take two minutes rest between sets, eventually decreasing the rest interval to a steady one minute. After completing the four months, you'll be transformed, amazed and amazing.

Weeks 1-2 (24 sets)

Exercise	Sets	Reps
Leg Raises	2	10
Sit-Ups	2	10
Squats	2	8-10
Stiff-Legged Deadlifts	2	8-10
Calf Raises	2	15-20
Bench Press	2	8-10
Chin-Ups (Lat Pulldowns)	2	8-10
Bent-Over Rows	2	8-10
Standing or Seated Press	2	8-10
DB Side Laterals	2	8-10
Curls	2	8-10
Lying Extensions	2	8-10

Weeks 3-6 (19 sets)

Exercise	Sets	Reps
Sit-Ups	2	15
Squats	3	8-12
Stiff-Legged Deadlifts	2	8-12
Bent-Over Rows	3	8-12
Upright Rows	2	8-12
Pushdowns	2	8-12
Wrist Curls	2	10-15
Calf Raises	3	10-15

Weeks 7-10 (35 sets)

Exercise	Sets	Reps
Leg Raises	3	20
Squats	4	10-15
Stiff-Legged Deadlifts	3	8-12
Deadlifts	2	6-10
Chin-Ups (Lat Pulldowns)	4	8-12
Shrugs	2	10-15
Standing or Seated Press	3	6-10
Curls	3	8-12
Lying Extensions	3	8-12
Wrist Curls	2	10-15
Reverse Curls	2	10-15
Seated Calf Raises	4	10-15

Weeks 11-16 (43 sets)

Exercise	Sets	Reps
Sit-Ups	2	20
Leg Raises	2	15
Squats	4	10-15
Leg Curls	3	8-12
Deadlifts	3	6-10
Bent-Over Rows	3	8-12
Chin-Ups (Lat Pulldowns)	2	8-12
Upright Rows	3	8-12
Standing or Seated Press	3	6-10
DB Side Laterals	2	8-12
Curls	3	8-12
Lying Extensions	3	8-12
Reverse Curls	2	8-12
Wrist Curls	3	10-15
Calf Raises	5	15-20

Full Body to Split-Body Transition Program

Ϋ Dumbbells, Barbell, Adjustable Bench, Power Rack, High Cable, Leg Curl

This routine takes the beginning weight trainer through a four-week bodybuilding program, starting gradually with an introduction to full-body training, slowly increasing the workout volume, intensity and variety, culminating with a graduation to intermediate split-body training by the fifth week.

Week 1

🕐 *45-60 minutes , 3 days per week*

Take two minutes rest between each set.

Exercise	Sets	Reps
Crunches	1	12
Leg Raises	1	12
Incline Press	1	12
Chin-Ups (Lat Pulldowns)	1	12
Bent-Over Rows	1	12
Pushdowns	1	12
Curls	1	12
Squats	1	15
Stiff-Legged Deadlifts	1	15

Weeks 2–4

🕐 *20-45 minutes , 3 days per week*

For these next three weeks, you'll reduce the rest periods to one minute between each set, and perform one additional set of each exercise each week, until you are completing four sets of each exercise by week four.

Exercise	Sets	Reps
Leg Raises	2-4	12
Sit-Ups	2-4	12
Bench Press	2-4	12, 10, 10, 8
Bent-Over Rows	2-4	8-10
Curls	2-4	8-10
Pushdowns	2-4	10-12
Squats	2-4	15
Calf Raises	2-4	15-20

Weeks 5+

🕐 *30-60 minutes , 3 days per week*

Starting with week five, you'll migrate from the full-body workout scheme of the past four weeks to a more advanced split-body routine—working your upper body in **Workout A** and the lower body in **Workout B**. Keep alternating between these workouts, three days per week, until you feel ready to move onto one of the dedicated split-body routines. After completing this program, you'll be conditioned to volume, intensity, variety, success and failure—graduating Weight Training 101.

Workout A (Upper Body)

Exercise	Sets	Reps
Bench Press	3-4	12, 10, 8
Chin-Ups (Lat Pulldowns)	3-4	10-12
One-Arm Row	3-4	8-10
Seated Press	3	8-10
DB Side Laterals	3	8-10
Curls	3-4	8-10
Close-Grip Bench Press	3-4	12

Workout B (Lower Body)

Exercise	Sets	Reps
Squats	4	12, 10, 8, 6
Stiff-Legged Deadlifts	3	10
Leg Curls	3-4	10-12
Calf Raises	4	To failure
Seated Calf Raises	4	To failure

Beginner's Barbell Workouts

Ψ Barbell, Bench, Power Rack

Here, we'll turn to an adaptation of the classic five sets of five reps system ("5x5"), popularized in the bodybuilding realm by Reg Park. During his bodybuilding reign in the 1950s and 1960s, Reg Park exemplified the perfect balance between aesthetic physique and phenomenal strength—this is what we are after here. Reg was 6'1" and weighed over 240lbs without the use of pharmaceutical enhancement. He was also the acknowledged inspiration for a kid from Austria—Arnold Schwarzenegger, so this is a good place to start.

This routine is comprised of heavy compound movements, performed with the 5x5 protocol. However, unlike the classic 5x5 routine from legendary strength coach Bill Starr, Reg Park's adaptation uses the first two sets as graduated warm-ups for sets 3-5 (this is also the adaptation used prominently by Mark Rippetoe today in the strength world).

To give you an example of how you should train using this system, let's assume you can bench press 100lbs for 5 reps (which should be about 90% of your one-rep max). Your first set would be at 60lbs for five reps (60%), and the second warm-up set of five reps would be 80lbs (80%). Sets 3-5 would be at 100lbs for five reps. Every exercise, other than calf work, follows this protocol. In this system, you train your arms and calves with higher reps for as much weight as you can handle in good form.

You'll perform this work three days per week, typically Monday, Wednesday and Friday, but any three days will suffice, as long as you provide a complete day of rest between each training session. Alternate between Workout A and Workout B each time you train.

Workout A

Exercise	Sets	Reps
Squats	5	5
Chin-Ups or Pull-Ups	5	5
Dips or Bench Press	5	5
Barbell Curls	2	10
Wrist Work	2	10
Calves	2	15-20

Workout B

Exercise	Sets	Reps
Front Squats	5	5
Rows	5	5
Standing Press	5	5
Deadlifts	3	5 (one work set)
Wrist Work	2	10
Calves	2	15-20

Intermediate Bodybuilding

This is where most spend the majority of their lifting career.

At the intermediate level of bodybuilding, the lifter has accumulated the necessary foundation of initial strength, balance and neuromuscular acclimation, in addition to the body's adaptation to volumes of hard work. At this point, we measure progress by weekly achievement, since workout-to-workout increases have largely dissipated.

Now it's time to dissect the workload of the physique into a more specific regimen and radiate the exercise variations outward, without neglecting the foundation of basic movement patterns. This is where we go beyond the simple two-way split routine of upper/lower body and introduce more complex split-training programs, in order to maintain the locomotion of adaptation.

Two-Way Split: Workout #1 (2 Days per Week)

🕐 *15-45 minutes*
🏋 *Dumbbells, Barbell, Bench, Power Rack*

For this workout, perform 1-3 sets of each exercise for 6-10 reps on upper body movements, and 10-20 reps on lower body exercises. Take 1-2 minutes rest between sets. Suggested workout days are Monday and Thursday, although you can change that to anything that fits your schedule—just try to keep two rest days between each workout.

Monday (Legs, Chest, Upper Back, Abs)

Exercise	Sets	Reps
Squats	1-3	10-20
Bench Press	1-3	6-10
Chin-Ups or Bent-Over Rows	1-3	6-10
Good Mornings	1-3	6-10
Calf Raises or Seated Raises	1-3	10-20
Wrist Curls	1-3	6-10
Crunches	1-3	10-20

Thursday (Lower Back, Shoulders, Arms, Abs)

Exercise	Sets	Reps
Sumo or Stiff-Legged Deadlift	1-3	10-20
Standing or Seated Press	1-3	6-10
DB Side Laterals	1-3	6-10
Curls	1-3	6-10
DB Side Bends	1-3	10-20

Two-Way Split: Workout #2
(2 Days per Week)

⏲ 30-45 minutes
Ⴤ Barbell, Bench, Power Rack, High Cable

If you have only an hour or two per week to train, yet still have dreams of building bigger muscles, fear not—if you give everything you've got for 30-45 minutes twice per week, this routine will get you there. If you manage to find another 30 minutes in the week, do it three times per week. Always alternate between **Workout A** and **Workout B** each training session. Both workouts include some direct abdominal work for your core, although the deadlifts and squats will provide their own indirect effect on that area.

Workout A (Hamstrings, Shoulders, Back, Triceps, Abs)

Exercise	Sets	Reps
Stiff-Legged Deadlift	1	15
	1	10
Standing or Seated Press	1	10
	1	6
Chin-Ups (Lat Pulldowns)	2	8-12
Pushdowns	2	6-10
Calf Raises	1	25
	1	20
Leg Raises	1	10-20

Workout B (Legs, Chest, Traps, Shoulders, Arms, Abs)

Exercise	Sets	Reps
Squats	1	15
	1	10
Bench Press	1	12
	1	8
Shrugs	1	15
	1	10
Seated Press	1	8
Chin-Ups (Lat Pulldowns)	2	6-10
Curls	1	10
	1	6
Seated Calf Raise	1	30
	1	25
Sit-Ups	1	15-20

Two-Way Split: Workout #3 (2 Days per Week)

🕐 *30-45 minutes*

🍸 *Barbells or Dumbbells, Adjustable Bench, Power Rack, High Cable*

This workout is similar to the previous one but adds a lot more volume in the same time frame, so you'll need to really push yourself to get it completed in the recommended time. Because it's so similar to traditional strength training workouts (albeit with more volume and less rest), many categorize this type of workout a *Power Bodybuilding* routine. Alternate between **Workout A** and **Workout B** each time you train and give it everything you've got.

Workout A (Chest, Back, Abs)

Exercise	Sets	Reps
Bench Press	4-5	15, 12, 10, 8, 6
Chin-Ups (Lat Pulldowns)	4-5	12, 10, 10, 10, 8, 8
Incline Press	4-5	10, 8, 6, 6, 6
Deadlifts	4-5	12, 10, 8, 6, 6
Crunches	2	15-20

Workout B (Legs, Arms, Abs)

Exercise	Sets	Reps
Squats	5	15, 12, 12, 10, 8
Stiff-Legged Deadlifts	5	12, 10, 8, 8, 8
Calf Raises	5	15-20
Curls	4	6-10
Pushdowns	4	10-12
Leg Raises	2	15-20

Two-Way Split: Workout #4 (3 Days per Week)

🕐 *30 minutes*
🏋 *Barbell, Bench, Power Rack*

The two workouts in this hypertrophy-based routine contain alternating pushing and pulling movements. Intermediates should perform 1-3 sets of each exercise. Keep the reps in the 6-8 range for best results. Try this routine three days per week, alternating between each workout.

Workout A (Shoulders, Traps, Arms, Abs)

Exercise	Sets	Reps
Standing or Seated Press	1-3	6-8
Shrugs	1-3	6-8
Close-Grip Bench Press	1-3	6-8
Curls	1-3	6-8
Sit-Ups or Crunches	1-3	12-15

Workout B (Back, Chest, Legs)

Exercise	Sets	Reps
Deadlifts	1-3	6-8
Bench Press	1-3	6-8
Bent-Over Row	1-3	6-8
Squats	1-3	6-8
Stiff-Legged/Romanian Deadlift	1-3	6-8
Calf Raises	1-3	6-8

　　　　　　　　　　Bodybuilding at Home

Two-Way Split: Workout #5 (3-5 Days per Week)

🕐 *45-60 minutes*

🍴 *Dumbbells, Barbell, Adjustable Bench, Power Rack, High Cable*

This training program is divided into upper and lower body workouts. You'll select one of the routines each workout, alternating between the two. You can perform this routine 3-5 days per week, based on your motivation, energy levels and recovery ability. For the first four weeks, perform two sets of each exercise—after that add an additional set and reduce your rest intervals from 2-3 minutes between sets to 1-2 minutes.

Upper Body Routine

Exercise	Sets	Reps
Standing or Seated Press	2-3	10-12
Chin-Ups (Lat Pulldowns)	2-3	10-12
Incline Press	2-3	10-12
Bent-Over DB Lateral Raises	2-3	10-12
Bench Press	2-3	10-12
Bent-Over Row	2-3	10-12
Pushdowns	2-3	10-12
Curls	2-3	10-12
DB Side Lateral Raises	2-3	10-12
Reverse Curls	2-3	10-12

Lower Body Routine

Exercise	Sets	Reps
Stiff-Legged Deadlift	2-3	12-15
Good Mornings	2-3	12-15
Front Squats	2-3	12-15
Lunges	2-3	12-15
Calf Raises	2-3	12-15
Leg Raises	2-3	15-20
Crunches	2-3	15-20

Two-Way Split: Workout #6 (4 Days per Week)

🕐 *45-60 minutes*
🍸 *Dumbbells, Barbell, Adjustable Bench, Power Rack*

In previous routines, you've seen how to split your body into two workouts and alternate between those each training day. Here it's the same protocol, except you'll double the frequency, performing each workout twice per week.

MON/THURS (Chest, Shoulders, Arms, Calves)

Exercise	Sets	Reps
Bench Press or Incline Press	5	6-12
Standing or Seated Press	4	6-12
DB Side Lateral Raises or Bent-Over DB Lateral Raises	3	8-12
Curls	3	8-12
Seated Extensions	3	8-12
Wrist Curls	2	10-15
Seated Calf Raises	3	10-20

TUES/FRI (Back, Legs, Abs)

Exercise	Sets	Reps
Bent-Over Rows	4	6-12
Chin-Ups (Lat Pulldowns)	3	To failure
Squats or Front Squats	5	6-12
Lunges or Reverse Lunges	3	10-15
Stiff-Legged Deadlifts	4	6-12
Calf Raises	3	10-20
Leg Raises or Crunches	3	15-20

Two-Way Split: Workout #7 (6 Days per Week)

🕐 *45-60 minutes*

🍸 *Dumbbells, Barbell, Adjustable Bench, Power Rack*

With this routine you'll be training six days per week, alternating between two different workouts. Sunday is for rest. Amen.

MON/WED/FRI (Abs, Chest, Shoulders, Back)

Exercise	Sets	Reps
Leg Raises	1	20
Bench Press or Incline Press	5	6-12
Seated Press	4	6-12
DB Side Lateral Raises	2	10-12
Chin-Ups (Lat Pulldowns)	3	To failure
Bent-Over Rows	3	6-12

TUES/THURS/SAT (Abs, Legs, Arms)

Exercise	Sets	Reps
Crunches	1	20
Squats or Front Squats	4	6-15
Stiff-Legged Deadlifts	4	8-12
Good Mornings	2	12-15
Curls	2	8-12
Seated Extensions	2	8-12
Wrist Curls	2	10-15
Standing or Seated Calf Raises	3	10-15

Three-Way Split: Workout #8
(3 Days per Week)

🕐 *15-30 minutes*
🍸 *Dumbbells, Barbell, Bench, Power Rack*

For this workout, perform 1-3 sets of each exercise for 6-10 reps on upper body movements, and 10-20 reps on lower body exercises. Take 1-2 minutes rest between sets. Suggested workout days are (surprise!) Monday, Wednesday and Friday, although you can change that to anything that fits your schedule—just try to keep one rest day between each training session.

Monday (Legs, Back)

Exercise	Sets	Reps
Squats	1-3	10-20
Stiff-Legged Deadlifts	1-3	10-20
Chin-Ups (Lat Pulldowns) or Bent-Over Rows	1-3	6-10

Wednesday (Abs, Calves, Arms)

Exercise	Sets	Reps
Crunches	1-3	10-20
DB Side Bends	1-3	10-20
Standing or Seated Calf Raises	1-3	10-20
Curls	1-3	6-10
Wrist Curls	1-3	6-10
DB Side Lateral Raises	1-3	6-10

Friday (Chest, Shoulders)

Exercise	Sets	Reps
Bench Press	1-3	6-10
Standing or Seated Press	1-3	6-10

Three-Way Split: Workout #9 (3 Days per Week)

🕐 *20-30 minutes*

🍴 *Barbell, Adjustable Bench, Power Rack, High Cable*

You aren't limited to dividing your bodybuilding program into two distinct workout sessions when training on a three day per week schedule. Here, we split the routine into three different workouts, each on their own day. This is a good power bodybuilding scheme if you can devote only about 30 minutes to each workout—now there are no excuses. Try it, work hard, and watch how it packs on the muscle.

Monday (Lower Back, Chest, Abs)

Exercise	Sets	Reps
Deadlifts	3	6
Incline Press	3	6
Weighted Crunches	3	12

Wednesday (Upper Back, Biceps, Calves, Abs)

Exercise	Sets	Reps
Chin-Ups (Lat Pulldowns)	3	To failure
Curls	2	6
Calf Raises	2	15
Crunches	1	To failure

Friday (Legs, Triceps, Shoulders, Calves)

Exercise	Sets	Reps
Squats	1	8
	2	To failure
Pushdowns or Dips	2	To failure
Seated Press	3	6
Seated Calf Raises	2	20

Three-Way Split: Workout #10
(6 Days per Week)

45-60 minutes
Dumbbells, Barbell, Adjustable Bench, Power Rack

Extending our last routine, here we add more frequency (now you are training six days per week), more volume within each workout, and increase the average rep range—therefore, you get more time to get through each workout.

MON/THURS (Abs, Chest, Shoulders, Triceps)

Exercise	Sets	Reps
Leg Raises	1	20
Bench Press or Incline Press	5	6-12
Seated Press	4	6-12
DB Side Lateral Raises	2	8-12
Seated Extensions or Close-Grip Bench Press	3	6-12
Reverse Wrist Curls	2	10-15

TUES/FRI (Abs, Upper Back, Biceps, Calves)

Exercise	Sets	Reps
Crunches	1	20
Chin-Ups (Lat Pulldowns)	4	To failure
Bent-Over Rows	4	8-12
Curls	3	8-12
Wrist Curls	2	10-15
Calf Raises	3	10-20

WED/SAT (Abs, Legs, Lower Back)

Exercise	Sets	Reps
Leg Raises	1	20
Squats or Front Squats	5	6-15
Stiff-Legged Deadlifts	4	6-12
Good Mornings	3	10-15
Seated Calf Raises	3	10-20

Four-Way Split: Workout #11
(4 Days per Week)

🕓 *60 minutes*

ᵞ *Dumbbells, Barbell, Adjustable Bench, Power Rack, High Cable*

Over the past twenty years, I've had good success with this four-day per week routine, training each muscle group directly once per week. Because you get only one shot every week to train each muscle group, you tend to stay focused—the last thing you want to do is go easy and have to wait another week to redeem yourself. Each workout should take you about one hour.

A couple notes about this routine:

- Hamstrings are trained on a separate day from thighs, because most people tend to either neglect or not put enough effort into them.

- If you start with Bench Press one week, then start with the Incline Press the next week. Keep rotating in that fashion—it helps to develop the entire chest symmetrically.

- The Monday and Friday workouts are pushing and pulling days, whereas Tuesday has pushing and squatting and Thursday is pulling and hinging movements. Again, balance is harmony.

MONDAY (Chest and Shoulders)

Exercise	Sets	Reps
Bench Press	5	6-12
Incline Press	5	6-12
Bent-Over DB Rear Laterals	3	8-12
Seated Press	5	6-12
DB Side Lateral Raises	3	8-12

TUESDAY (Thighs, Calves and Abs)

Exercise	Sets	Reps
Squats	5	6-12
Front Squats or Hack Squats	5	6-12
Seated Calf Raises	4	8-20
Standing Calf Raises	4	8-20
Leg Raises	3	15-20

THURSDAY (Back, Traps, Hamstrings)

Exercise	Sets	Reps
Chin-Ups (Lat Pulldowns)	5	To failure
Bent-Over Rows	5	6-12
Shrugs	5	6-12
Stiff-Legged Deadlifts	5	6-12

FRIDAY (Arms and Abs)

Exercise	Sets	Reps
Curls or Drag Curls	4	8-12
Reverse Curls	4	8-12
Close-Grip Bench Press	5	6-12
Seated Extensions	3	8-12
Pushdowns or Dips	3	To failure
Crunches	3	15-20

Five-Way Split: Workout #12 (5 Days per Week)

🕐 *30-40 minutes*

🍸 *Dumbbells, Barbell, Adjustable Bench, Power Rack*

A lot of people like training Monday through Friday after work, taking the weekend off. If you're going to be a weekday warrior, do it right and train one muscle group on each day, for about 30-40 minutes (more for large muscle groups, less for smaller ones). Here's one example of how you might structure this type of routine.

For the inexperienced, there is a method to the (seeming) madness here. First, while your energy reserves are built up from a weekend of high-carb eating (and maybe drinking?), you'll want to hit a large muscle group like the back. After that initial day of pulling movements, the next day you should push, so chest comes next on the menu. Legs are reserved for midweek and will drain most of your remaining energy (see, it really is *hump day*). Therefore, Thursday is relatively easy compared to the previous day's effort, and Friday is for arms, because every Friday is International Arms Day. Seriously, by Friday you'll be longing to get out of the gym and collapse into the weekend, so some smaller muscles like arms, calves and abs seems about right.

MONDAY (Back, Abs)

Exercise	Sets	Reps
Deadlifts	3	6
Chin-Ups (Lat Pulldowns)	3	To failure
Bent-Over Rows	3	8-10
Crunches	2	To failure

TUESDAY (Chest)

Exercise	Sets	Reps
Bench Press	4	6-8
Incline Press	3	8-10
Guillotine Press	3	12

WEDNESDAY (Legs, Abs)

Exercise	Sets	Reps
Squats or Front Squats	5	8-12
Romanian Deadlifts or Stiff-Legged Deadlifts	4	8-12
Leg Raises	3	15-20

THURSDAY (Shoulders, Traps)

Exercise	Sets	Reps
Standing or Seated Press	4	8-12
DB Side Lateral Raises	3	10-12
Bent-Over DB Rear Laterals	3	10-12
Shrugs	4	6-12

FRIDAY (Arms, Calves, Abs)

Exercise	Sets	Reps
Curls or Close-Grip Pull-Ups	4	8-12
Reverse Curls	2	10-12
Close-Grip Bench Press	4	6-10
Wrist Curls	2	12-15
Standing Calf Raises	3	12-15
Seated Calf Raises	3	12-15
Leg Raises	2	15-20

SATURDAY & SUNDAY

God rested one day—here you get two.

Advanced Bodybuilding

Most never reach this level.

Why? Because moving beyond intermediate levels of bodybuilding, much like any other strength-oriented activity, requires the identification of weaknesses, long-range planning to eliminate those weaknesses, rigorous execution of the plan, and advanced overload techniques.

In other words, you need to discover that you have to do so much less (simplify!), but do all of it so much better (technique, intensity, planning, execution). It's here that home gyms really let you focus—maybe that's why advanced weight trainers eventually migrate back to the home gym or the small, hardcore gyms that remain.

Although the intricacies of periodization-based training, as applied to bodybuilding are well beyond the scope of this book, it may be useful to present some bodybuilding workouts that incorporate advanced overload techniques that you can add to those existing intermediate workouts. This will provide you a glimpse of the world of advanced bodybuilding. (If you are at the advanced level, my book *Supermen: Building Maximum Muscle for a Lifetime* contains extensive information about advanced bodybuilding training, including over 200 advanced workouts.)

Advanced Overload Training (AOT)

AOT techniques have a taxing effect on the neuromuscular system—this is more than likely to exceed a beginner or intermediate trainer's capacity for adaptation. Overreaching and overtraining are likely results here. Tread carefully.

Although a complete treatment of AOT techniques is beyond the scope of this book (and is covered in my other books), here's a list of these advanced adaptation-inducing methods for the advanced trainer:

- 21s
- Addition Sets
- Alternating Sets
- Ascending Sets
- Burns
- Cheating
- Compound Sets
- Down the Rack
- Drop Sets
- Fixed Time Sets
- Forced Reps
- German Volume Training (GVT)
- Giant Sets
- Halves
- Negatives
- Partials
- Pre-Exhaustion
- Pyramids
- Rep Targeting
- Rest-Pause
- Russian Ladders
- Same Weight Progression
- Static Holds
- Supersets

From this list of AOT techniques, you can incorporate one or more of them into a training program. Here's one example.

Pre-Exhaustion

🕐 *60 minutes*
🏋 *Dumbbells and/or Barbell*

The idea here is to "pre-exhaust" a muscle group by performing a single-joint movement for the area, quickly followed by a multi-joint movement for that same area. Here's a sample workout using this technique throughout.

Exercise	Sets	Reps
Squat	1	20
Deadlift	1	20
DB Fly	3	15
Bench Press	3	10
Pullover	3	15
Bent-Over Row	3	10
Front Raise	3	15
Standing or Seated Press	3	10
Standing Calf Raise	3	15
Side Bends	1	15
Crunches	3	20

• • • •

Full-body workouts are not just for beginners. You can extend full-body workouts into the realm of advanced training by adding advanced overload techniques, as I've described previously, or by simply manipulating time. Here's an example.

Full-Body Advanced 8x8 Workout

⏱ 30-60 minutes
Ⴤ Dumbbells, Barbell, Bench, Power Rack

Vince Gironda, the legendary bodybuilder and trainer from the 1950s was a huge advocate of full-body, three-times per week training, especially for advanced trainers. One of the intensity techniques he employed was the reduction in rest times between sets. In the workout below, instead of adding more weight to the bar, reduce the rest intervals. Start with 45-60 seconds rest between sets. Every time you make it through the workout, getting all 8 reps for 8 sets, cut the rest period by 5 seconds. Start this routine with weights that are about 60% of your normal 8-rep max (with typical 1-2 minute rest periods). Once you can get your rest intervals down to 30 seconds, that's the time to add more weight and start the process over. You can also rotate exercises, as you see fit. At some point, you may see Jesus here, especially during the squats. Good luck.

3 Days per Week

Exercise	Sets	Reps
Bench Press	8	8
Chins (Lat Pulldowns)	8	8
Triceps Extensions	8	8
Barbell Curl	8	8
Lateral Raises	8	8
Squats	8	8
Calf Raises	8	8

Adapting Workouts for the Home Gym

There are endless books, articles and videos detailing various bodybuilding workouts you can perform. Typically, these workouts require equipment, particularly machines found in commercial gyms. This section describes how you can adapt these workouts to the equipment you have in your home gym.

Substituting Dumbbells for Barbells

In almost all cases, you can substitute the dumbbell-based version of an exercise in place of the barbell version. Here's some examples.

Barbell Exercise	Dumbbell Versions
Squats	Squats, Goblet Squats, Split Squats
Bent-Over Row	Bench Rows, One-Arm Row
Military Press	DB Press, Arnold Press, W-Press
Shrugs	DB Shrugs, Bench Shrugs, Seated Shrugs

There are a few barbell-based exercises that become difficult, from a performance perspective, when using dumbbells, such as cleans. However, this is where kettlebells can offer some effective alternatives.

What about using Barbells in place of Dumbbells?

When we start talking about using a barbell as a substitute for dumbbell exercises, our landscape of hypertrophy-based exercises starts to narrow. Most of this is due to the unilateral, three-dimensional movement that dumbbells allow, such as flys for the chest. Lesson here—if you intend to be a bodybuilder, you need dumbbells.

Substituting Free Weights for Machines

For this situation, we look back to the men (and don't' forget the women!) who forged themselves in during the pre-1950s era and the exercises they used, before the machines took over. Those early machines were designed to improve the ease, stress and results for various movements. Ease and stress, yes—but results, not so much (stress is for good and not just evil purposes!). Most of the free weight substitutions are obvious, but obvious to me may not equate to everyone reading this, so I'll be explicit. Below, the machine exercise is listed first, followed by the common free weight exercises that equal, and often, surpass the machines.

Chest Machines

Chest Press: Barbell/DB Press (flat, incline, decline), Dips

Pec Dec: DB Flyes (flat, incline, decline)

Cable Crossover: DB Flyes (flat, incline, decline)

Back Machines

Lat Pulldown: Chins, Pull-Ups

Seated Cable Row: One-Arm DB Row

Supported T-Bar Row: Barbell T-Bar Row

Row: Bent-Over Barbell Row

Pullover: Barbell or DB Pullover

Low Back Extension: Good Mornings

Shoulder Machines

Shoulder Press: Barbell Military Press, DB Press, Arnold Press

Lateral Raise: DB Lateral Raise

Arm Machines

Preacher Curl: Barbell and DB Preacher Curl

Pushdowns: Close-Grip Bench Press, Reverse-Grip Bench Press

Triceps Extension: Barbell and DB Extensions

Leg Machines

Leg Press: Squat, Front Squat

Hack Squat: Barbell Hack Squat, Front Squat

Leg Extension: Sissy Squat

Lying/Standing/Seated Leg Curl: Romanian Deadlift, Stiff-Leg Deadlift

Adductor/Abductor: Wide-Stance Squats

Calf Machines

Standing Calf Raise: Barbell Calf Raise, One-Leg DB Calf Raise

Seated Calf Raise: Seated Barbell or DB Calf Raise

Integrating Cardio into Your Workout Routines

Lifting progressively heavier weights is an anabolic activity. The body adapts to this stress by growing stronger and larger muscles to handle the consistent load. Conversely, cardiovascular activity ("cardio") is an inherently catabolic activity, albeit one that does play an important role in overall heath and fat loss. The trick becomes how to balance and intertwine the two, seemingly conflicting activities into a cohesive training plan.

Luckily, others have already shown us the way.

Bodybuilders of the 1940s through the 1960s didn't engage in much direct cardio work, as we define it today (stationary bike, elliptical, or stair climbing). However, they did perform lots of what we would call 'active rest', things orthogonal to weight training, such as hand balancing, gymnastics and yes, manual labor. All of these activities tended to burn any excess calories that would have been stored as fat. It also made a clear statement to the body that it was expected to perform physical activity of any sort.

While the 1970s ushered in the era of running, jogging and other activities on the extreme of the cardiovascular duration spectrum, former Mr. America Clarence Bass was writing about his success with simple walking, typically every evening as a post-dinner activity with his wife.

As the 1980s, through the next thirty years, plastered us with Jane Fonda and the aerobics generation, followed by the extreme foolishness of The Biggest Loser™, we saw a continual pattern emerge of cardiovascular duration, intense, daily physical punishment (what Dan John would call "smoking"), and yelling. More than often, these forms of "cardio" are detrimental, both physically and mentally.

Lucky for us, recently Marty Gallagher has once again conjured Ocaam's Razor into the world of physical transformation and reminded us that remarkable changes can be achieved with un-remarkable methods. Marty and his clients engage in (surprise!) walking to shed body fat and build conditioning. Not just a stroll in the park, but rather a progressively (there's that word again) harder walk up the mountainous nature trails that abound behind his central Pennsylvania home.

So, Clarence and Marty's fused message is that integrating something as simple as walking into your daily routine—something that our ancestors had no choice but to follow for survival—is two-thirds of the common-sense trifecta "secret" to health, strength, and fitness. Extreme methods and yelling not required. When we as a species stopped walking out of necessity and survival, and sat down in the comfort of air-conditioning (as Mark Rippetoe so often laments), we set ourselves on this course of physical degradation.

Coming directly back to our topic—how do we integrate cardio into our workouts?—we'll use the wisdom of Bass and Gallagher for the simplest approach that just plain works:

- Don't perform cardio with your weight lifting sessions. Let the body learn that it needs to adapt solely to progressively heavier loads during training sessions.

- Walk. More importantly, integrate walking into your life. I especially like Bass's approach here of the walking ritual after dinner. This has many benefits, beyond involving your spouse, children or pets. The natural world displays innumerous species going for long walks after eating a meal. Watch what a dog does, given a bowl of food and an open yard. That's a good lesson from man's best friend. Although Clarence and Marty walk outside—and I highly suggest you do the same—you can also do this indoors on a treadmill if necessary. Not as pleasant or maybe productive, but still can be effective.

- What if you need to perform cardio indoors, due to climate, weather or time of day? Or you don't have much time in your daily schedule? This is where the spectacular results of Professor Izumi Tabata come into play. By leveraging your stationary bike, rower, treadmill, elliptical, kettlebells or, for those masochists, the barbell front squat (in the power rack, please!) along with Tabata-style cardio training (twenty seconds of intense work were followed by ten seconds of rest, repeated continually for four minutes), those gut-wrenching four minutes could change the shape of your life.

Thank You

Thank you for buying this book. I hope that you've found the information beneficial and a good value.

I have a free deal for you.

If you liked this book and think it was helpful, then please write a sentence or two about this book on Amazon or whatever place you ordered from (write an honest reaction—whether positive, negative or neutral). Do that, and send me an email at books@runningdeersoftware.com telling me where I can read your feedback and I'll email back to you my **bonus report listing the recommended equipment by manufacturer and model** you should consider for every type of item listed in this book. There are specific recommendations for budget, economy and luxury spending for every category, so you'll find the best option for your wallet. I keep this list updated all the time, because things do change over time.

Additionally, if you email me about a recommendation for a piece of equipment that I currently don't recommend, I evaluate it and update my list based on your recommendation, I'll ship to you all of my other books free of charge. If you help me, I'll take care of you.

Other Books by Craig Cecil

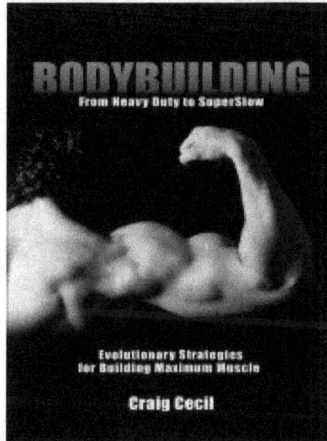

Bodybuilding: From Heavy Duty to SuperSlow

Bodybuilding: From Heavy Duty to SuperSlow takes you through the evolution of bodybuilding training, from early 20th century circus strongmen to the latest muscle-building techniques of today. Learn how to harness these concepts to build muscle faster than you thought possible.

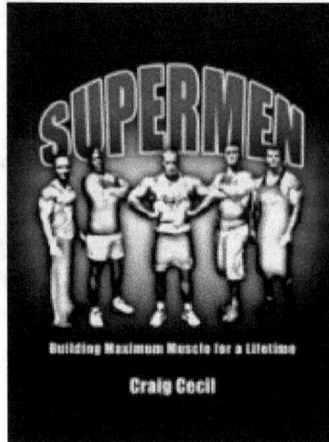

Supermen: Building Maximum Muscle for a Lifetime

Supermen: Building Maximum Muscle for a Lifetime presents a weightlifting system for intermediate to advanced weight trainers that maximize the muscular development of an individual, while creating a complete, balanced and symmetrical physique. This book will save you years of trial-and-error in the gym and provide you with decades of weight training insights. It's a book for the rest of us—those with average genetics, strong minds and stronger hearts. More significantly, it represents a long-term plan for lifting weights wisely throughout your life while building and maintaining significant muscle mass.

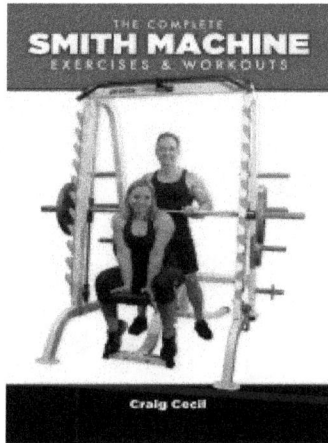

The Complete Smith Machine: Exercises & Workouts

The Complete Smith Machine: Exercises & Workouts is the most comprehensive resource ever written about the most popular exercise machine in the world. Whether you use a Smith Machine at home, the gym, or are thinking about buying one, this book contains all the information you'll need to use and master this versatile piece of weight training equipment.

Software for your Computer (PC or Mac)

If you liked this book, you may be interested in software, which supports the material you just read.

Running Deer Software (www.runningdeersoftware.com) provides low-cost spreadsheet and browser-based software for workout tracking and preparation, exercise selection, fitness testing, and diet analysis.

MuscleCALC
Weightlifting workout log and analysis system (spreadsheet).

FitnessCALC
Fitness assessment testing and tracking (spreadsheet).

Exercise Genie
Exercise encyclopedia and workout builder (spreadsheet).

Diet Genie
Food database and nutritional analysis system (spreadsheet).

Exercise Gambler
Random workout generation using a fun slot-machine game (browser app).

About the Author

Craig Cecil has been involved in sports and the science of exercise since his days of high school athletics in baseball, through his collegiate career in NCAA Track & Field, to his devotion to weightlifting and bodybuilding pursuits over the past 20 years. During that time, Craig has trained with professional athletes, as well as multitudes of dedicated, ordinary individuals just wanting to build lean, muscular body weight. Craig is a member of the National Strength & Conditioning Association and holds an MBA from Loyola University of Maryland.

www.ingramcontent.com/pod-product-compliance
Lightning Source LLC
Chambersburg PA
CBHW062158270326
41930CB00009B/1570